THE
BODY CLOCK GUIDE
Using **Traditional Chinese Medicine**
for Prevention and Healthcare

By Zhang Jiaofei & Wang Jing

Better Link Press

This book is edited and designed by the Editorial Committee of *Cultural China* series.

Text: Zhang Jiaofei, Wang Jing
Translation: Cao Jianxin
Photos: Liu Shenghui, Ding Guoxing
Design: Wang Wei

Assistant Editor: Hou Weiting
Copy Editor: Kirstin Mattson
Editors: Zhang Yicong, Wu Yuezhou
Editorial Director: Zhang Yicong

Senior Consultants: Sun Yong, Wu Ying, Yang Xinci
Managing Director and Publisher: Wang Youbu

ISBN: 978-1-60220-120-0

Address any comments about *The Body Clock Guide: Using Traditional Chinese Medicine for Prevention and Healthcare* to:

Better Link Press
99 Park Ave
New York, NY 10016
USA

or

Shanghai Press and Publishing Development Co., Ltd.
F 7 Donghu Road, Shanghai, China (200031)
Email: comments_betterlinkpress@hotmail.com

Printed in China by Shanghai Donnelley Printing Co., Ltd.

3 5 7 9 10 8 6 4

Contents

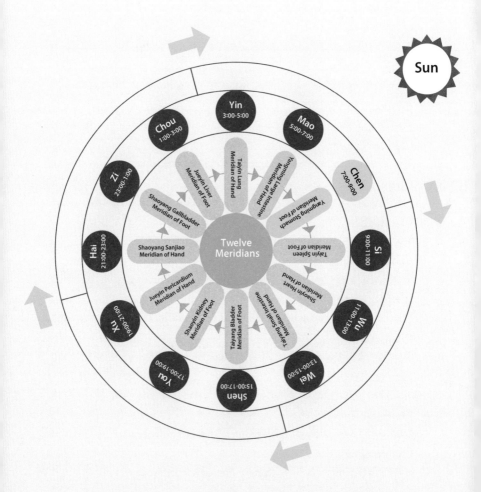

Relationship between the Twelve Periods of Day and Meridians

Preface

Let Mother Nature Guide You to Optimal Health

The concept of living one's life in harmony with Mother Nature is an ancient one that still has great value today. We can find meaningful advice in *Yellow Emperor's Inner Canon*, an ancient medical text that has served as a basis for traditional Chinese medicine (TCM) for more than two millennia. This classic has been handed down from generation to generation, and its rules about living according to the seasons, the time of day, and other natural principles are all you need to prevent and cure diseases, and bring about your own optimal health.

As we know a year features the changes of spring, summer, autumn and winter. In Chinese philosophy a day is characterized by changes of twelve periods of two hours each. In addition, the environment is marked by differences of dampness and dryness while the climate features differences of cold and heat.

We naturally follow the changes of Mother Nature with many of our existing habits and practices of work and rest. For example when the weather turns from hot to cold, people put on more clothes, and they turn to hot food in winter and cold food in summer. When the sun ascends, people also get up and begin to move around, and when it descends, people go to sleep. While seemingly quite ordinary, these habits adhere to the laws of nature.

There are other ways to follow the natural progress of a day that may be less familiar to most of us. Each of the twelve periods of the day, as defined in ancient Chinese texts, corresponds to one of the twelve regular meridians and collaterals in the human body. These are pathways through which qi (vital energy) and blood circulate, and through which the organs, limbs and body exterior are connected. The meridian, and the internal organ with which it is associated, are at their prime for a specific two-hour period each day.

At its peak period, most of the body's energy and blood run through the specific meridian concerned. For example at Wu Time (11 a.m. to 1 p.m.) the Heart Meridian is in its prime. Ample energy and blood serve to further adjust the function of the organ related to the meridian, in this case the heart. When the function of the internal organ is reinforced, there will be a high efficiency of bio-chemical metabolism.

In addition to correlating with different meridians and organs, the periods of the day, and of the year, are also connected with changes of yin and yang. Central to the practice of TCM, yin and yang are the two fundamental principles or forces in the universe. Yin reaches its peak at midnight and in winter, while yang energy is strongest at midday and in summer.

Zi Time (11 p.m. to 1 a.m.), for example, is marked by complete quietness in Mother Nature, as yin, which reaches its peak and then begins to decline, is exchanged with yang. At this time the Gallbladder Meridian is in its prime, hence making it the best time to recuperate the gallbladder and protect yang. It is important to rest in bed at this time, otherwise it will affect the generation of the gallbladder's Shaoyang energy, leading to a variety of ill effects, including a bitter taste in the mouth, looking grey, feeling hesitant, and experiencing pain such as aches in the heart and intercostal region.

On the other hand at Wu Time (11 a.m. to 1 p.m.) as the sun is hottest, yang is the most vigorous in the world around us. As the Heart Meridian is in its prime, a short nap helps recuperate yin, without which we might have too much heart-heat, canker sores, agitation and insomnia among other symptoms.

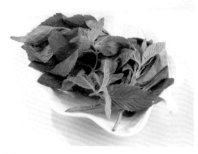

Mint

Traditional Chinese medicine attaches great importance to acupoint therapy. By massaging or tapping acupoints, we can clear our meridians, promote blood circulation and help remove and cure diseases. Again it is important to follow the body clock, as it is most effective to treat a specific meridian when it is at its peak.

We must pay attention to natural laws when choosing our food as well. All food comes from nature and is assigned different traits in TCM. These include the "four energies" (hot, warm, cold and cool plus neutral) and the "five tastes" (sweet, sour, bitter, salty, spicy/pungent). These refer to the inherent qualities of the food rather than their actual temperature or flavors, although these are often closely related. If we understand the nature of food we can use diet to recuperate health and prevent disease.

For instance mutton, pepper and shrimp tend to be marked

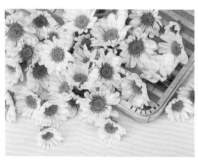

Wild Chrysanthemum

by yang, and therefore serve to strengthen yang. Those who have a yang-deficiency should incorporate foods such as these in their diet for better health. Food choice also relates to the time of day. As yang is growing during the morning, it is best not to eat or drink overly

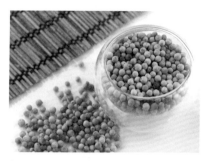

Pepper

cold food (such as iced juices) because this will cause the rising yang energy and blood to cool and stagnate.

Integrating diet with natural laws also extends to the environment in which we live. Some areas in southern China are very damp, resulting in the habit of eating spicy food because this can get rid of the cold and dampness in the body to prevent diseases. In the north, where it is quite dry, the people's yang is fairly strong and they eat less spicy food. And as stated previously, in winter, people enjoy eating hot food, while the opposite is true for summer. When we follow these natural preferences we follow Mother Nature, and keep our bodies in harmony.

This book takes you back to the basic concepts of healthcare expounded in *Yellow Emperor's Inner Canon*, and gives practical advice on how to apply these concepts in the modern world. Each of the book's twelve chapters corresponds to a period of time, which in turn relates to a specific meridian and its associated internal organ. You will find easy-to-follow tips on choosing the right massage, food and exercise for the time of day, and for your own particular health needs.

We need not invest in complicated equipment, drugs or procedures to recuperate our bodies and reach optimal health. The answer lies simply in Mother Nature. Following the body's own clock will uncover the secret of healthcare, and help you make the choices right for your own body, leading to a happy, healthy and long life.

Chapter One

Zi Time (11 p.m. to 1 a.m.)
Gallbladder Meridian in Its Prime

Zi Time refers to the hours around midnight when all things remain still, which can be compared to the winter of a year. At this time your body must focus on "storing up" while you quietly wait for the arrival of daytime. This is when the Shaoyang Gallbladder Meridian of Foot (Gallbladder Meridian) begins to work, and the smooth operation of internal organs in your body depends on the gallbladder.

According to the classic Chinese text, *Yellow Emperor's Inner Canon*, at midnight, yin begins to wane while yang starts to wax. When yin and yang are alternated, a new cycle begins. At Zi Time most people are sleeping, and sleep is exactly what is needed to help nourish and develop yang. Those who do not sleep at Zi Time face a myriad of future troubles. The sleeping state does not mean that the body is completely "turned off" because the Shaoyang Gallbladder Meridian of Foot is on its "night duty."

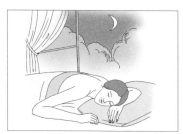

Sound Sleep Helps Develop Yang
Sleep can not only replenish stamina and restore strength, but also nourish the gallbladder and protect yang. It is important to nap between 11a.m. and 1 p.m., even if one has to forego a meal, as well as to go to sleep before Zi Time.

Ordinarily you may feel sleepy a short while after supper. However you will feel more alert and also hungry around 11 p.m. In fact the activity of the Gallbladder Meridian is at its prime at this moment. After a day's work, bile needs to be metabolized, and it is only when you are asleep that your bile can complete this process of metabolism.

Yellow Emperor's Inner Canon points out that the normal operation of internal organs depends on the development of bile, which in turn depends on sleep quality during Zi Time. If sleep quality can be ensured at Zi Time, the gallbladder will function normally.

Undertaking activity during this time when yin and yang alternate, or going to sleep after midnight, will use up yin and prevent your yang from being developed. This weakens the protection of your body and hampers the smooth operation of energy and blood all over your body.

In these cases the symptoms may be a bitter taste in the mouth, frequent sighing, and pain in the chest and costal cartilages when you turn your body slightly. More severe symptoms include dullness of the facial skin, and feeling as if you are covered with dust and cannot be washed clean. You may feel that the skin all over your body is not fine any longer, and your feet are hot on the outside.

This is caused by the deficiency of Shaoyang energy, the type of yang energy that flows in this meridian. These symptoms indicate that your gallbladder has a problem and you should take steps toward recuperation or consult a doctor.

Sleeping at Zi Time Is Vital

Yellow Emperor's Inner Canon states that if a day is compared to a year, Zi Time would be equivalent to winter. In winter the earth is frozen and most animals slow down or even hibernate. Likewise our body also goes to sleep around midnight.

Zi Time is the exact turning point of yin and yang alternation. Yin reaches its peak and yang gradually develops from its valley, as the body enters a new cycle. With the alteration of night and day, our view of the sky changes, with the moon visible at night and the sun shining during the day. Therefore we say that the moon and the sun belong to yin and yang respectively.

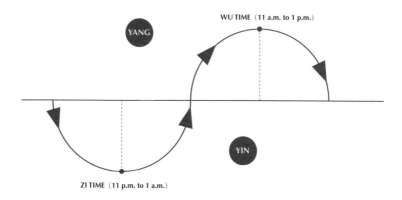

The Change of Yin and Yang at Zi Time
At Zi Time, which is the turning point of yin and yang alternation, yin reaches its peak while yang develops from its valley and waxes gradually.

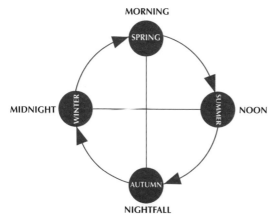

The Four Times of Day and the Four Seasons in a Year
Zi Time is the time of day that is equivalent to the season of winter. Just as animals hibernate in winter, people will sleep at Zi Time.

When the moon is in the sky, we should sleep, "storing up," and nourishing yin and protecting yang. During the day we should move about vigorously, especially going outdoors to bathe ourselves in the sunshine. If you choose to sleep in the day, your yang will be frustrated and you will violate a basic natural law, diminishing your opportunity for good health. Therefore sleeping at Zi Time conforms to the way of nature and the change of yin and yang. In this way we can protect yin and yang in our body, and in doing so, protect our health.

Late Night Activity Harms Health

Burning the midnight oil, i.e. undertaking activities late at night, will exhaust the vital essence in your body, trigger gallbladder-related diseases, and affect your decision-making capacity.

At Zi Time, the energy and blood of your liver and gallbladder collaterals, most of which are used to support metabolism, reach their peak. If too much energy and blood are diverted to the brain, limbs, intestines and stomach due to late-night activity, the waste in your body cannot be eliminated in a timely manner, and fresh energy and blood cannot be generated smoothly.

Therefore if you often burn the midnight oil, your bile cannot

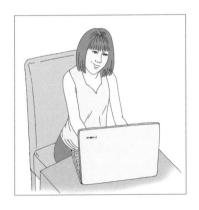

Burning the Midnight Oil Prevents Yang from Developing

The underdevelopment of Shaoyang energy will lead to such phenomena as livid face-color, hard breathing and confusion, and may hinder your thoughts and judgment.

metabolize in time, and may thicken and crystallize, causing gallstones in the long run. If bile overflows, you will feel a bitter taste in mouth, your face will become discolored, and you will suffer from migraines. You may even feel depressed and dispirited all day. Moreover other parts of your body will also ache accordingly, e.g. sciatica, hyperplasia of the mammary glands, and costal cartilage pain.

Although sleeping late and undertaking late-night activities may seem insignificant, they can do huge harm to your body. Although the harm may not be apparent when you are young and full of energy and blood, it will manifest as you age.

Burning the midnight oil can not only bring about diseases but also affect thinking and judgment, because it prevents the energy of gallbladder from developing. Insufficient energy of the gallbladder will prevent you from being decisive. *Yellow Emperor's Inner Canon* also says that sufficient gallbladder energy in the body will prevent exogenous pathogenic factors from invading, thus strengthening health.

In contrast insufficient gallbladder energy will bring about timidity and indecision. If you go to sleep before 11 p.m., your bile will be normally metabolized and your gallbladder can function as it should. This will allow you to think soundly and make resolute decisions, as well as maintain a glowing appearance and a high spirit in the daytime.

Night Snacking Is Not Advisable

Some people say that it is hard for a hungry man to go to sleep, and that a person with a full stomach will sleep soundly. However if you go to sleep with a full stomach, your digestive system will still work when you are asleep. As the movement of the intestines and stomach needs to be nourished by yang, this will use up the yang energy that has just developed.

In the long run this will prevent the Shaoyang energy in your gallbladder from developing normally. Your Gallbladder Meridian will not flow correctly, the secretion of bile will decrease, and gallbladder function will decline. The most obvious symptom of harm to gallbladder energy is oily hair. This is because the oil you have ingested cannot be broken down effectively, and therefore is discharged via the hair.

If people who work overtime have to snack at night to keep up their strength, it is best to take some light porridge or soup, which can not only be digested and absorbed easily but is also nourishing. However, as stated earlier, for the best health, night snacking is not advisable.

For the gallbladder, breakfast is a must. Early morning is exactly the time when the Stomach Meridian works. As long as the stomach is in motion, bile is secreted. If the secreted bile cannot interact with digested nutrition from food, and runs in an empty state for a long time, gallstones will occur. Those who skip or have a late breakfast face a higher risk of gallbladder problems.

"Combing" Can Get Rid of All Worries

Yellow Emperor's Inner Canon says that when women/men are at the age of 42/48 respectively, the yang in their body declines, slowly turning their hair grey. Grey hair usually occurs on temples at the very beginning. Nowadays, due to living habits or other factors, the hair of many young people turns grey prematurely. This is caused by insufficient energy and blood in their body. The radical treatment of this symptom depends on the Gallbladder Meridian.

Insufficient energy and blood of the Gallbladder Meridian leads to premature grey hair. If this meridian has no vitality, gallbladder energy will not develop and the energy and blood in the body will become insufficient. When the hair cannot absorb enough nutrition, it will turn dry and grey. On the contrary, if you

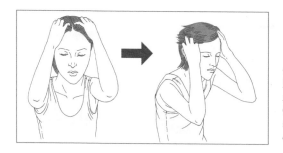

Grasping a correct head-combing method can dredge Gallbladder Meridian and prevent and cure diseases.

go to sleep before 11 p.m., your gallbladder energy will develop, the energy and blood of your Gallbladder Meridian will become sufficient, and your hair will absorb the required nutrition and will not turn grey naturally.

The best way of preventing premature grey hair is to "comb" your hair, and a correct method can clear your Gallbladder Meridian. "Combing" is a technique derived from traditional Chinese medicine, and does not refer to using an actual comb. Instead you should comb your hair with the pads of all fingers, from the front hairline to the rear, from the center to both sides, 300 times a day, with a moderate force. Gently press your scalp with your fingers, until your scalp becomes slightly hot.

The human head is covered with many meridians, including the Gallbladder Meridian, Stomach Meridian and Bladder Meridian. If your gallbladder has some problem, you will feel an ache when you comb a corresponding point. In particular the sides of the head are covered with Gallbladder Meridian points. If you feel any ache at a point when you are combing, that means a block has occurred at that point, and you should rub and knead it repeatedly until it is cleared.

Clearing your head helps keep your whole body clear. Combing your head regularly can get rid of various diseases, not only premature greying, hair loss and dry hair, but also helping to resist and prevent colds. For the elderly this method can improve such symptoms as dizziness and insufficient blood supply to the brain, and prevent senile dementia.

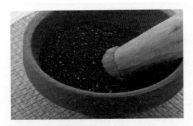

Black Sesame

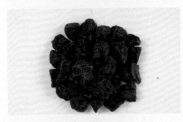

Polygonum Multiflorum

Two Methods for Nourishing Hair
1. Sesame
Sesame can nourish and produce hair as well as enrich the blood. A small spoon of fried sesame can be taken every day, or a bowl of sesame paste can be eaten every morning.

2. Hair Blackening Tea
Ingredients: 40 g polygonum multiflorum, 20 g dried rehmannia root, 100 g Chinese dates, 20 g Chinese wolfberry, 40 g wild chrysanthemum, 20 g rock sugar.
Preparation: Put together in boiling water to create tea.

How to Exercise the Gallbladder Meridian

How should we maintain the normal function of the gallbladder? The most direct way is to tap the Gallbladder Meridian every day.

Tapping is an ancient technique based on traditional Chinese medicine, using the hand or simple instruments to tap on certain points in the body to enable the flow of qi or energy through the body. For the gallbladder, tapping focuses on the Shaoyang Gallbladder Meridian of Foot, which extends from the head to the sole of the foot.

This meridian's route is quite complicated, starting from the outer eye corner, going upward to the frontal angle, then going downward. It again travels upward after passing the rear of the ear, going to the upper side of the eyebrow after passing the forehead, then returning to the rear of the ear. It goes along the side of the neck before reaching the Shaoyang Sanjiao Meridian of Hand, receding on the shoulder, crossing the Shaoyang

Sanjiao Meridian of Hand, and going forward and entering the supraclavicular fossa.

The Gallbladder Meridian has many branches.

- Ear branch: It separates at the back of the ear, enters the ear, goes out and passes the front of the ear and reaches the rear of the outer eye corner.

- Outer canthus branch: It separates from the outer eye corner, goes downward and reaches the Daying point at the mandible, meets the Shaoyang Sanjiao Meridian of Hand, and passes the lower part of the eye socket. It then reaches the angle of the mandible and neck, meets the foregoing branch at the supraclavicular fossa, then goes downward and enters the body cavity. After crossing the diaphragm, it contacts the liver and gallbladder, then goes along the waist rib, passes the lower abdomen, and horizontally enters the Huantiao point of the hip joint.

- Supraclavicular fossa branch: It goes downward from the supraclavicular fossa to the armpit, goes along the lateral of the thorax, then passes the hypochondrium. It proceeds downward to the hip joint and meets the preceding branch, going downward and along the outside of the thigh, knee and shin. It then goes directly downward to the front of the tip of the lateral malleolus, along the instep and enters the outside of the fourth toe.

- Instep branch: It separates from the instep, moves forward, and goes out from the lateral of the big toe. It then goes back, crosses the toenail, distributes itself behind the nail of the big toe, and meets the Jueyin Liver Meridian of Foot.

To stimulate your Gallbladder Meridian, you can frequently tap both flanks of your thigh, your costal cartilages and both sides of your head. You can tap your Gallbladder Meridian at any time and any place.

For example, while standing, place your hands on both flanks of the thigh. The place where the tip of your middle finger rests is

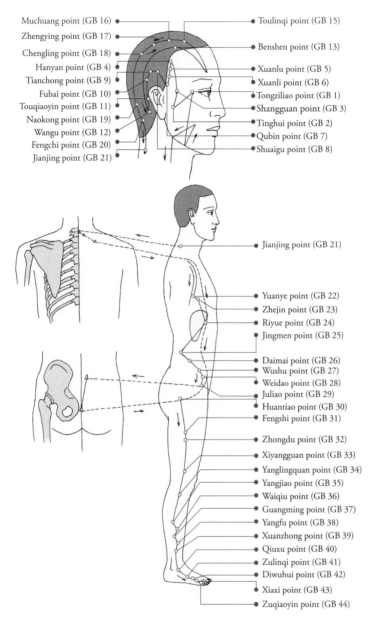

Muchuang point (GB 16)
Zhengying point (GB 17)
Chengling point (GB 18)
Hanyan point (GB 4)
Tianchong point (GB 9)
Fubai point (GB 10)
Touqiaoyin point (GB 11)
Naokong point (GB 19)
Wangu point (GB 12)
Fengchi point (GB 20)
Jianjing point (GB 21)

Toulinqi point (GB 15)
Benshen point (GB 13)
Xuanlu point (GB 5)
Xuanli point (GB 6)
Tongziliao point (GB 1)
Shangguan point (GB 3)
Tinghui point (GB 2)
Qubin point (GB 7)
Shuaigu point (GB 8)

Jianjing point (GB 21)

Yuanye point (GB 22)
Zhejin point (GB 23)
Riyue point (GB 24)
Jingmen point (GB 25)

Daimai point (GB 26)
Wushu point (GB 27)
Weidao point (GB 28)
Juliao point (GB 29)
Huantiao point (GB 30)
Fengshi point (GB 31)

Zhongdu point (GB 32)
Xiyangguan point (GB 33)
Yanglingquan point (GB 34)
Yangjiao point (GB 35)
Waiqiu point (GB 36)
Guangming point (GB 37)
Yangfu point (GB 38)
Xuanzhong point (GB 39)
Qiuxu point (GB 40)
Zulinqi point (GB 41)
Diwuhui point (GB 42)
Xiaxi point (GB 43)
Zuqiaoyin point (GB 44)

Shaoyang Gallbladder Meridian of Foot

the Fengshi point, from which wind can enter your body the most easily. While pressing this place, you will often feel it is hard. Therefore when you pat it you should squat slightly. Tapping both flanks with your hands can achieve the effect of exercising the meridian. After being tapped the skin may appear black and blue, which indicates you have already patted away any stasis of wind. The disappearance of bruising indicates that your Gallbladder Meridian has been cleared.

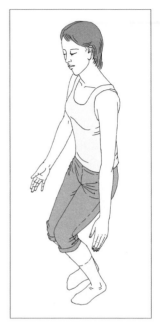

Tap thigh of ten to stimulate Gallbladder Meridian.

Cure Various Eye Diseases and Headache: Rub and Knead Tongziliao Point and Guangming Point

As the starting point of the Gallbladder Meridian, the Tongziliao point is located at the depression beside the eye corner. The Guangming point is located 5 cun (a cun is a traditional and individualized measurement defined as the distance across the uppermost joint of your thumb) above the tip of the lateral malleolus. Often pressing and rubbing these two points can cure myopia, cataract, glaucoma and other eye diseases.

Cure Indigestion, Hangover and Stomach Discomfort: Rub and Knead Shuaigu Point

The Shuaigu point is located about 1.5 cun above the tip of ear. The word "gu" in the name of this point refers to cereal; therefore this point is definitely related to eating and drinking. If you eat too much, feel nauseated, feel like vomiting or have a headache after drinking, just press and rub this point.

19

Lose Weight and Cure Constipation, Migraine, Hyperplasia of Mammary Glands, Gynecopathy and Prostate: Tap Daimai Point
The Daimai point is located on both sides of the waist at the level of the navel. It can be hard to find the Daimai point of obese people. The best way is to relax your body while lying flat, and tap the place under the ribs and above the hipbones, more than 200 times each round, on both sides. Young people can tap this place frequently to stimulate weight loss, while women can tap this point often to prevent hyperplasia of the mammary glands and relieve painful menstruation. In the elderly, regular tapping here will reinforce movement of the large intestine and cure constipation.

Prevent and Cure Cholecystitis and Gallstones: Tap Zhongdu Point and Rub and Knead Riyue Point
Frequently tapping the Zhongdu point (located on the outside of the thigh and 2 cun below the Fengshi point) can clear stasis due to the inability to discharge toxins in the liver. The Riyue point is located in the seventh intercostal space under the nipple, 4 cun away from the anterior median line and on the inside line of the nipple. Massaging this point can also help clear the Gallbladder Meridian and effectively prevent and cure cholecystitis (inflammation of the gallbladder) and gallstones.

Chapter Two

Chou Time (1 a.m. to 3 a.m.)
Liver Meridian in Its Prime

Chou Time witnesses the darkness before dawn and anticipates sunlight on the horizon. At this time yin falls while yang rises. Tranquility begins to embrace activity, weeding through the old to bring forth the start of a new day.

During Chou Time work moves from the Gallbladder Meridian to the Jueyin Liver Meridian of Foot (the Liver Meridian), since the liver operates the flow of energy and blood at this time. The liver plays the role of storing blood and adjusting blood volume. According to *Yellow Emperor's Inner Canon*, people need more blood when they move around. In order to meet these needs, the liver provides blood storage, with energy and blood running through the meridian. As the body stands still, it requires less blood, with a great deal of blood being stored in the liver. This prepares the body for the day's activity.

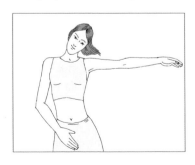

Human Movement Attributed to Blood Circulation

People need more blood when they move around. The liver provides blood to meet these needs. Circulation of energy and blood comes first.

The liver is the main internal organ for detoxification, which is its main function. Every day we come into contact with and absorb many toxic substances, which are harmful and must be dispersed. Otherwise they will propagate quickly to harm our health.

How can we get rid of these toxic substances? This is completely the work of the liver. First the liver decomposes toxic substances absorbed by the intestines or produced by other parts of the body. Then it turns them into harmless substances and secretes them into the bile or blood before they are finally discharged from the body.

This may sound simple but the process is complex. Ample energy and blood are required by the liver for detoxification. The liver, after working during the previous day, also needs to renew old blood with fresh blood.

At 2 or 3 a.m., energy and blood flow through liver to complete the process of blood metabolism. If you do not rest at this time, your blood has to run directly through the meridian, making blood metabolism impossible in the liver. If this occurs on a regular basis, the liver becomes over-burdened in its work, leading to illness.

At the same time the liver is also in charge of the tendons, and without ample blood to nourish the tendons, they will lose their elasticity.

Sound Sleep Needed at Chou Time

For liver recuperation, high-quality sleep is a must. In addition, mental activity is not advisable before sleep, as too much strain on the brain will obstruct the generation of yang. This not only affects the quality of sleep but also makes you particularly exhausted in the daytime.

According to *Yellow Emperor's Inner Canon*, people will

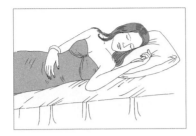

Blood Stored in Liver When Body Is Still
Less blood is needed when the body is not in motion. At this time, lots of blood is stored in the liver.

have ample energy and blood in the liver if they stay in bed for a rest. This will nourish the eyes, feet, hands and fingers. Energy and blood will complete the process of metabolism if one rests or stays in a still state and relaxes.

Therefore liver recuperation is possible not only at night but also in the daytime if you take time off for a short nap. A short rest after supper can also recuperate the liver and get rid of tiredness. According to the view of traditional Chinese medicine, it is better to go to sleep before Zi Time so the liver and gallbladder can be well recuperated.

Thinking is closely associated with the liver, so ample energy in the liver can lead to quick reasoning and reaction, greatly enhancing work efficiency. Otherwise people will be slow to respond, failing to make a success of things.

According to *Yellow Emperor's Inner Canon*, yang energy in the human body follows the principle, "Generation in spring, growth in summer, contraction in autumn and storage in winter." People should follow a natural rhythm in their clothing, food, sleep, activity and feelings.

We must adapt ourselves to the four seasons so that the generation of the body correlates with the changes of Mother Nature. *Yellow Emperor's Inner Canon* holds that spring is the best season for recuperating the liver. Corresponding to spring, the liver is in charge of generation, and both show signs of activity and vigor. Additionally the liver corresponds to wood in the Five Elements, a theory that is one of the bases of traditional Chinese

Liver's Relationship to Four Seasons and Other Important TCM Concepts

	Liver	Points of Attention
Four Seasons	Spring	All things grow in spring. People should go to bed and get up early, keep their hair and clothes loose in the morning, and walk for relaxation, since these are conducive to protecting the liver.
Five Elements	Wood	The liver is linked with wood, because it resembles grass and wood that grow in spring, a time during which liver function is quite active.
Five Flavors	Sour	The liver is fond of sour. Eating an appropriate amount of sour food is conducive to recuperating the liver. However eating too much sour food will lead to coarse and contracted muscles as well as dry and split lips.
Five Colors	Green	The liver is fond of green. Eating more green food can effectively reduce pressure on the liver and gallbladder and adjust their functions. For instance, lychee, plum, celery, water-spinach and mung beans are good for reducing liver-heat.
Five Entities	Tendon	The liver is in charge of the tendons, which rely on energy and blood in the liver for nourishment. Ample energy and blood in the liver can lead to strong tendons, while inadequate energy and blood in the liver will result in a lack of nourishment for the tendons, hence giving rise to hand and foot tremors, numb limbs and difficulty in limb extension, etc.
Five Sentiments	Anger	Anger harms the liver. Excessive anger is apt to result in the adverse rise of liver energy followed by the adverse rise of blood. An angry person often suffers from a red face and ears, headache, dizziness and even blood-vomiting and coma, etc.
Five Cereals	Wheat	Wheat and polished round-grained rice are marked by the effect of contraction. Frequently eating porridge of wheat and polished round-grained rice serves to recuperate the liver, protect the blood, nourish yin and reduce heat.

medical practice. In spring, trees sprout, getting ready to bear fruit in summer and autumn.

The most important function of the liver is adjusting the flow of energy and blood all over the body. This allows internal organs

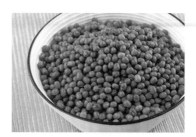

Mung Beans

to be well nourished, reinforcing our ability to resist fatigue. However too much liver energy in the spring is not good, since it is apt to lead to a "damp" and tired spleen and stomach, making these organs operate abnormally and suffer from inadequate energy of their own. Consequently people will feel tired and dizzy among other symptoms.

Protecting Eyesight Related to Recuperating Liver

A myriad of electronic gadgets, including TVs, computers and mobile phones, make our lives more colorful. However eyesight may become blurry and eyes may become dry when sitting in front of TVs and computers every day. Over time eyesight will gradually become worse; this is because our eyes can no longer stand the strain.

While *Yellow Emperor's Inner Canon* is an ancient text it has relevant advice: "Reading too long harms the liver and sitting too long harms bones," and "Blood goes to the liver when one stays in bed, and one can see clearly when there is ample blood in the liver."

Here we see cause and effect. Sitting for a long time before the television and computer consumes lots of blood in the liver, and the timely backflow of blood into the liver will be affected if one stays sleepless overnight. Consumption of blood in the liver without any replenishment leads to problems of the eyes as well as various other symptoms. Therefore staying in bed for a rest is

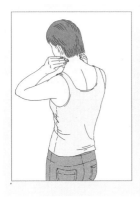

Massage Neck
Rub the neck with the palms for about three to five minutes, until the neck feels slightly warm, since this serves to promote blood circulation in the area. Normal blood circulation around the neck can bring more energy and blood to the head, whose blood-supply can directly influence the eyes. Therefore rubbing the neck in this way is good for improving the blood-supply of eyes as well as the entire brain.

necessary to bring about replenishment and nourish the eyes. This is exactly why it is so important that the liver should be nourished first.

According to *Yellow Emperor's Inner Canon*, under normal situations, the liver provides blood and yin essence to nourish our eyes, enabling us to clearly distinguish various colors. Therefore spirited eyes stand for ample blood in the liver, while dull eyes signify the loss of blood in the liver. As people become old, they naturally suffer from the loss of blood in the liver. Their eyesight will become blurred if their eyes are not nourished adequately by blood in the liver.

In order to avoid excessive use of the eyes and prevent fatigue, people should close their eyes for a short rest once every hour, or look into the distance to give their eyes appropriate rest.

Female Health Based on the Liver

Some women radiate good health with firm and glowing skin, sleek and shining hair, high spirits, quick reactions and agile movement. On the other hand some women have sallow, thin skin and dry hair, and exhibit absent-mindedness and labored movement. Why are there such big differences? This is due to the

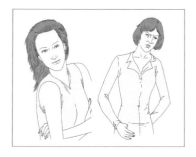

Desirable and Undesirable Liver Functions

When the liver functions optimally, women look rosy and beautiful.

When the liver is not operating properly, women suffer from the loss of energy and blood, with unsteady moods and hot tempers.

lack of blood in the liver.

The liver chiefly contains blood, the essence of human beings. This is particularly the case with women. Important stages in the female life cycle, starting from monthly menstruation during puberty to pregnancy, delivery and breast-feeding, require a lot of energy and blood. Only the "blood bank" (the liver) offers inexhaustible blood. The lack of blood in this "blood bank" leads to irregular menstruation and abnormal leucorrhoea, and even infertility if it becomes serious.

As we have learned, anger harms the liver. In women, anger can even harm the mammary gland and womb. The Liver Meridian passes through the female breasts, so if there are problems with the liver, it can lead to chest-fullness, breast-distension and breast pain. The womb is related to the liver, which is in charge of tendons. Due to its elasticity, the womb can change size through contraction. When experiencing anger, women must pay attention to changes in their bodies, particularly their breasts. Adjusting one's mood is fundamental in dealing with these effects on health.

Give Vent to Anger

In this world no one is free from getting angry. Anger takes place often and has varied causes, such as failure to be promoted and to get a raise, the disobedience of children, and quarrels with others.

When getting angry, one feels the loss of control and may find it difficult to eat. In serious cases this can lead to feeling dizzy and fullness in the chest along with abdominal pain.

According to *Yellow Emperor's Inner Canon*, anger harms the liver, excessive joy harms the heart, over-thinking harms the spleen, sorrow harms the lungs, and terror harms the kidneys.

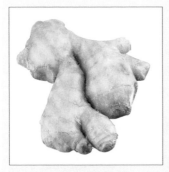

Ginger

Glossy Ganoderma Chicken Soup—Food as Medicine for Liver and Nerves Among the different kinds of poultry, chicken is particularly associated with the liver. Therefore chicken soup serves to nourish blood and yang in the liver very well. Delicious chicken soup with glossy ganoderma (a type of mushroom) not only tonifies the liver and calms nerves, but also benefits people suffering from insomnia resulting from neurosism.

Ingredients: Three-yellow chicken of about 2000 g (this is a specialty chicken in China, and can be substituted with any free-range chicken), 2 glossy ganodermas, 1 Chinese onion, ginger.

Preparation: Wash the chicken, cut the ginger into pieces, and put them together into a cookpot. Cut the Chinese onion into fine pieces, and add, along with the glossy ganodermas, to the other ingredients in the pot. Add an appropriate amount of water and boil under high heat. After 10 minutes take away the froth on the surface. Then boil on a low flame for an additional hour. Add salt to taste and boil for 15 minutes under medium heat.

The liver chiefly sorts out vital energy. Anger causes the adverse rise of liver energy, which runs wildly in the body and harms other organs. Liver energy works against the spleen, which can make the stomach distended. Liver energy also works against the stomach, which leads to hiccups, making it difficult to eat. There will be blood-vomiting if it is serious. Therefore to protect the liver, people must try not to be angry.

Some introverted people, particularly girls in many cultures, never vent their anger. Consequently liver energy, which cannot be discharged, goes to the costal region through the Liver Meridian to affect the breasts. Gradually there will be cyclomastopathy (fibrocystic disease).

In attempting to find a remedy the best way is to cry to discharge all the feeling. Crying is also a kind of detoxification. Since depression is gone afterward, there will be no harm to one's health. Of course one should not cry too much, because sorrow can negatively impact the lungs.

Liver energy should be marked by smoothness and comfort. Tenderness leads to desirable blood circulation whereas depression and anger cause an adverse rise of liver energy. It is dangerous if anger is kept inside, therefore finding a constructive way to deal with one's anger is a type of healthcare.

Chinese Leeks—Best for Liver Recuperation

Apart from a good sleep, people can make use of certain foods to recuperate the liver. Among the many kinds of food, which is the best? None other than Chinese leeks in spring.

As stated by Li Shizhen in the classic 16th century text, *Compendium of Materia Medica*, "Chinese leek-leaves are hot and their roots are warm in nature, with the same function. Raw

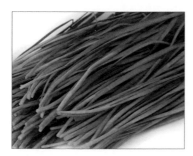

Chinese Leeks
Chinese leeks fall into the lily family of perennial herbs, with seeds and leaves taken as medicine. Chinese leeks serve to tonify the stomach, raise spirits, stop sweating, nourish the kidneys, and reinforce yang and sperm.

Chinese leeks serve to liven blood and fried Chinese leeks serve to replenish vital energy, hence being conducive to the liver." This points to the restorative properties of leeks on liver function.

In spring when all things grow, Chinese leeks are best for recuperating the yang of the liver. Cold air still remains to some extent in spring, so the yang in the body should be protected. Because of their mild and warm nature, Chinese leeks serve to tonify yang; reinforce liver, spleen and stomach functions; protect yang in the body; and strengthen the body's resistance.

Also according to *Compendium of Materia Medica*, "Chinese leeks taste good in spring, but are smelly in summer. Eating too many Chinese leeks would lead to unclear mentality and blurred eyesight. It is a taboo to eat them after drinking liquor." This means that one should pay attention to the season and amount when eating Chinese leeks. Eating too much can result in nosebleeds and even bleeding hemorrhoids among other conditions.

Despite their advantages, people must keep certain contraindications in mind when eating Chinese leeks. They are not suitable for those suffering from oral problems, aphtha, dry or sore throat, heat in the palm and sole, as well as sweating during sleep. Moreover pregnant women should avoid or only eat a small amount of Chinese leeks in order to prevent the movement of the fetus causing pain in the lower abdomen due to internal heat.

How to Exercise the Liver Meridian

The Jueyin Liver Meridian of Foot is the major meridian for adjusting liver functions. In daily life recuperating and exercising this meridian can adjust mood in addition to energizing blood and generating sperm.

The Jueyin Liver Meridian of Foot starts from the edge of the second joint of the big toe, and then travels across the point one cun ahead of the interior ankle, the point eight cun above the ankle, the inside of the knee, the inside of the thigh, and around the groin until it reaches the abdomen via the liver and gallbladder. Traveling across the diaphragm, it is divided into two lines under the eyes, one convenes the Baihui point (on top of the head) with the Governing Vessel (*Du Mai*) the other ends at the lips.

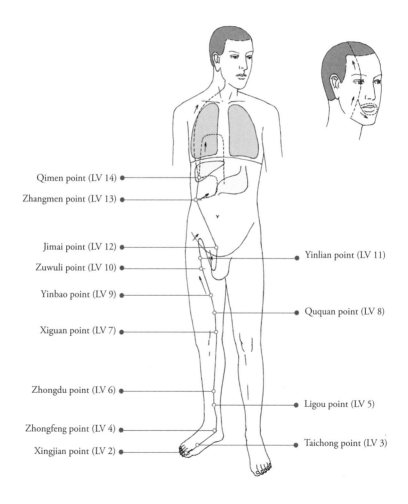

Qimen point (LV 14)

Zhangmen point (LV 13)

Jimai point (LV 12)

Zuwuli point (LV 10)

Yinbao point (LV 9)

Xiguan point (LV 7)

Zhongdu point (LV 6)

Zhongfeng point (LV 4)

Xingjian point (LV 2)

Yinlian point (LV 11)

Ququan point (LV 8)

Ligou point (LV 5)

Taichong point (LV 3)

Jueyin Liver Meridian of Foot

Massages for clearing the liver, once mastered, can adjust mood and bring about joy if you suffer from emotional upset. The focus lies in the areas of the liver and gallbladder, so as to stimulate these organs. In the course of massage, pinching can be applied, moving the fingers along while pinching. Attention should be paid to the force exerted by the fingers. This is excellent for clearing the liver to smooth vital energy, especially with regard to people who often suffer from depression.

Adjust Functions of Five Internal Organs: Rub and Knead Zhangmen Point

The Zhangmen point is a vital point of the Liver Meridian, serving as the gate to the internal organs. It is situated at the lower edge of the ribs. If you let your arms hang naturally alongside your body and then lift your hands with elbows bent, the Zhangmen point will be right under the elbow joint.

With arms akimbo, use your thumbs to rub and knead this point gently once every day for three minutes. Make sure that you don't rub and knead it when hungry, tired or within one hour after a meal to prevent the internal organ from being harmed. Rubbing and kneading the Zhangmen point can modify liver function smoothly and the functions of TCM's five internal organs will be strengthened accordingly.

Detoxification: Rub and Knead Taichong Point

Deserving its recognition as the number one acupoint in the human body, the Taichong point lies at a spot four centimeters above the sole between the big toe and second toe. Mostly this point is rubbed and kneaded when unhealthy qi and substances need to be discharged from the body. Since it is the original acupoint of the liver, rubbing and kneading it can enhance the effect of detoxification.

Some people often feel dizzy and tired. This is due to the weakness of liver functions and the inadequacy of energy and blood supplied by the liver to the heart. According to *Yellow*

Emperor's Inner Canon, wood generates fire; the liver is associated with wood while the heart is associated with fire. Inadequate wood leads to weak fire. Therefore the Taichong point should often be rubbed and kneaded in support of the liver.

The best method is to immerse the feet in hot water every evening, because hot water can stimulate the energy and blood of the feet, producing better results. Use two thumbs (or index and middle finger) to push, rub and knead slowly and forcefully forward to the Xingjian point, the second major point of the Liver Meridian. In this way two major acupoints can be stimulated at the same time. Additionally you should massage your feet, with each foot pushed, rubbed and kneaded for five minutes.

Push and Rub Costal Region

Press, push and rub the space between ribs from under the armpit to the chest, and repeat 30 times. The costal region refers to the lower chest ribs and the costal margins on either side of where the liver, gallbladder and pancreas are located. Pushing and rubbing the region frequently serve to reinforce liver functions as well as recuperate and protect the liver.

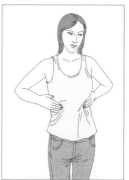

Exercise Outdoors

Frequently doing outdoor physical exercise to a proper extent is an optimal way to protect the liver. Physical exercise can promote air exchange and blood circulation, speed up metabolism and clear liver energy.

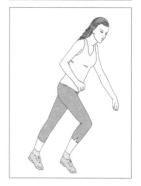

Keep a Sound Mentality

Try to be calm, joyful, optimistic

and outgoing, with a balanced frame of mind. Any kind of anger and depression, if persisting for a long time, leads to liver problems.

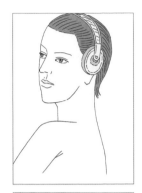

Excessive Alcohol Not Advisable

There is a limit to the alcoholic metabolism of the liver, and excessive amounts will be harmful to the liver.

Laws of Diet

The liver plays a key role in human metabolism, bile generation, detoxification, immunity, heat generation and adjustment of water and electrolytes. Too many drinks and too much food or frequent hunger can all lead to problems with liver functions or abnormal bile secretion. You should have three well-balanced meals a day, paying attention to the ratio of protein, fat, sugar, vitamin, minerals and water.

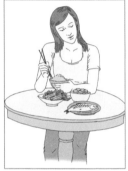

Drink Sufficient Water

As with eating, drinking water should also be regulated according to a fixed time and fixed amount. This can promote blood circulation, reinforce the vigor of liver cells, benefit liver recuperation and discharge waste.

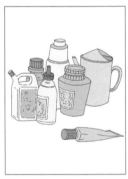

Avoid Toxins

In daily life, try to avoid contact with toxic substances, and avoid or be cautious in taking medicine harmful to the liver. This includes those containing lead, mercury, arsenic, benzene, aflatoxin and some other kinds of medicine (e.g. tranquilizers), since they can cause necrosis of liver cells to varying degrees.

Chapter Three

Yin Time (3 a.m. to 5 a.m.)
Lung Meridian in Its Prime

At Yin Time the Taiyin Lung Meridian of Hand (Lung Meridian) takes over from the Liver Meridian. The body changes from a static state and prepares for a more active one, thus requiring fresh energy and blood. At this time the lung plays its important role to balance the energy and blood all over the body.

According to *Yellow Emperor's Inner Canon*, the lung is equivalent to the "prime minister" of the five internal organs, assisting the heart ("sovereign") in nurturing the body. Therefore the lung plays a prominent role among the five internal organs.

At Yin Time (from 3 a.m. to 5 a.m.), night and day alternate, and the energy in the heavens and on earth turns from yin to yang. At this time energy and blood from all over the body flow into the Lung Meridian. The activity of this meridian becomes vigorous, transporting fresh blood stored in the liver to various blood vessels. This allows the energy, blood and fluid to be distributed all over the body, the internal organs are nourished, the hair is moisturized, and fluid goes downward to the bladder to ease urination. All of these actions help the body prepare for the arrival of a new day.

The lung is performing the duty of "balancing all" during this period, redistributing energy and blood all over the body. When the lung is performing this function of distribution, it must not

Symptoms of Light Sleep

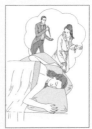 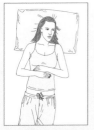 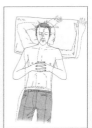 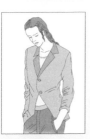

Remaining awake all night.	Tending to wake in the middle of the night, and having difficulty going to sleep again.	Often dreaming, and being able to remember the dreams after waking up.	Remaining listless and sullen in the daytime; working inefficiently.

be disturbed. Otherwise it would have to send more energy and blood to the activated organ, thus causing the uneven distribution of energy and blood, which could seriously harm the body.

Therefore the lung "hates" those who stay up until dawn and are active at Yin Time. To enable the lung to work normally, various organs are best brought into a state of dormancy at Yin Time.

Sound Sleep Helps Redistribute Energy and Blood

When the lung deploys energy and blood all over the body, one should be in a state of a sound sleep. Only when our body is in a thorough state of dormancy can the lung distribute energy and blood evenly.

According to the natural rhythm of the human body, people enter the best state of sleep 40 minutes after falling asleep. If you go to bed after 11 p.m., it may be very hard for you to sleep. This is because your brain is too excited due to yang in your body that has begun to develop itself.

Even if you do sleep, you will always be in a state of light sleep, during which you can be awakened easily or feel that you are dreaming at all times. Your internal organs are not completely in a state of rest, the adjustment function of the lung is impaired, and energy and blood cannot be distributed reasonably. After waking up the next morning you will feel tired all over the body as well as fuzzy-headed, so that working efficiency declines considerably.

How can we judge whether we are in a state of deep or light sleep? Deep sleepers usually go to sleep rapidly, rarely wake up at night, and can go to sleep again very soon even after waking. They rarely dream and often forget what they have dreamed after waking up. Deep sleepers often keep a sober mind and work efficiently in the daytime. Light sleepers are the opposite. Then how can we enter the state of deep sleep? It is most helpful to go to bed between 10 p.m. and 10:30 p.m. every day.

Breathing Exercises Promote Good Sleep

As we have learned, the lung is in charge of energy all over the body. At Yin Time, the Lung Meridian is in its prime, redistributing energy and blood all over the body, and therefore, people generally sleep very soundly at this time. If you wake up after midnight you may not go to sleep any longer. In particular, when you wake up at 3 a.m. or 4 a.m., this indicates that your lung energy is insufficient and your energy and blood are deficient.

These two are related, as according to TCM, "energy is the governor of blood." Energy and blood function, decline and stagnate at the same time. If lung energy is insufficient, the lung becomes powerless when distributing energy and blood. The blood also loses its driving force, and has difficulty in reaching every area of the body. Since energy and blood nurture the soul, the soul can become uneasy without the nourishment of energy

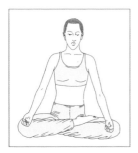

Breathing exercises are recommended when unable to sleep again after waking up at Yin Time.

and blood, leading to insomnia or premature wake-up.

Interruption of sleep is often a signal of insufficient energy and blood. The best cure is breathing exercises. If you cannot go to sleep, get up and put on clothes, and sit cross-legged facing south, just like a monk in meditation. Then put your clenched hands on your bent knees, with both eyes closed slightly. Move your tongue up and down in your mouth, touching the inside and outside of your teeth and gums to stimulate the generation of saliva.

According to traditional Chinese medicine, saliva and blood have the same source, originating from the essence of diet, and they produce and influence each other. Therefore insufficient energy and blood often lead to deficient saliva. In turn excessive loss of saliva often leads to loss of energy and blood. Sufficient energy and blood, and the balance between yin and yang, result in sound sleep and disappearance of diseases.

By exercising themselves in this way, people with weak energy and blood can achieve a good effect on their health, not only generating energy and blood but also benefiting the lung and protecting the kidney. Partaking of breathing exercises when one cannot go to sleep again after waking up at Yin Time can both promote sleep and nourish the body. People suffering from insomnia should give this a try.

Exercises in Bed Also Promote Health

It is important to do exercises in a timely and appropriate way, instead of randomly. Exercises can be modified to suit one's fitness level. For example it is not suitable for people with poor heart function to do exercises in early morning. However they can do exercises in bed to achieve the goal of health preservation.

As we have seen, early morning is when yang develops in the body. Taking a rest at this time can prevent interruptions of yang generation. Conversely doing outdoor exercises too early in the morning can prematurely consume yang and impair one's health. Moreover, in most locations, the sun has not yet risen and it is usually cold at Yin Time. Resisting the cold would consume considerable yang, which has just been generated. In addition, when the sun has not arisen, foul air on the ground goes upward. Exercises can accelerate breathing, and inhaling this air would also impair health.

People with a poor physical condition have insufficient energy and blood in their body. If they wake up at 4 a.m. or 5 a.m., it is very hard for them to go to sleep again. If they then get up and do outdoor exercises, some of their already insufficient energy and blood would be used to support various internal organs, and the burden on the heart would increase considerably. They could face serious health risks and even death under such circumstances.

What is the best time for getting up? It is generally acknowledged that getting up after 7 a.m. is the most appropriate. And what if we wake early in the morning? We can lie in bed with closed eyes. As yang rises in the early morning, lying still can sedate one's mind and nourish yang; sufficient yang prevents the body from being invaded by diseases. In addition to lying still, some light exercises in bed can be performed.

Comb Hair with Fingers

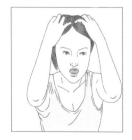

"Combing," or running your stretched fingers through your hair from front to back, promotes the cycle of energy and blood in the head, and also prevents hair loss.

Rub or Tap Outer Ear

Gently rub and knead the helix (outermost rim of the outer ear) with both hands until it becomes hot. Or tap the helix 100 times with your hands, starting from about 10–15 cm away and applying gentle force. Tapping the points covering the ears can not only foster movement of energy and blood but also activate kidney energy and normalize hearing.

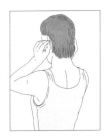

Rotate Eyes

Rotating your eyes, clockwise and anticlockwise for about one minute, exercises the eye muscles, and adds luster and spirit to the eyes.

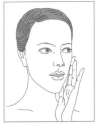

Click Teeth

Calm your mind, with your mouth and lips closed tightly. Relax your whole body and gently click the upper and lower teeth rhythmically for about 100 times. This can achieve the effect of reinforcing the teeth and promoting salivation.

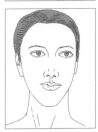

Massage Navel

Overlap your hands, palms facing your stomach, and gently massage the navel clockwise for three minutes. The navel is surrounded by vital acupoints such as the Guanyuan and Qihai points. This exercise can elevate mood and nourish vitality.

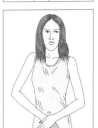

Withdraw Abdomen and Lift Rear

Repeatedly drawing in the abdomen and lifting the anal muscles can help in preventing and curing hemorrhoids.

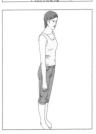

Turn Your Body

Turning your body to the left and right for one minute while lying in bed can exercise your spine and the muscles of your waist.

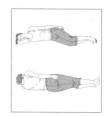

Rub Center of the Sole

The center of the sole of the foot is where the Yongquan point of the Kidney Meridian is located. The palm is where the Laogong point is located. Therefore massaging your sole with your palm (100 times is recommended) makes yin and yang embrace each other. This achieves the effect of tonifying your kidneys and reinforcing your heart.

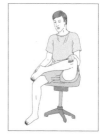

Avoid Being Excessively Cool in Summer

Lungs are quite fragile, and are susceptible to harm. Both internal and external cold can impair their function, while keeping warm can nourish the lungs.

The birth and death of all things can be attributed to yang, which is the essence of life. Human growth and the generation of body fluid depend on yang. Therefore we must learn how to nourish our yang.

When we are asleep, our energy and blood flows slowly and our body temperature drops slowly as well. At this time yang forms a protective layer on the body's surface to prevent pathogens from invading. In general this layer of yang cannot be destroyed when we are asleep. However if the window is open for ventilation or the air-conditioner is on, and there is not sufficient covering, a great deal yang will be consumed to resist the cold. This means that the protection layer of yang will be destroyed, the body will lose its screen, and the cold will invade our body through the skin.

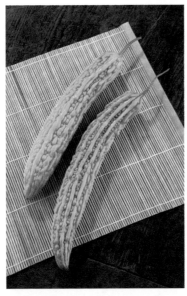
Bitter Gourd

When external pathogenic factors attack through the mouth, nose, skin and hair, our delicate lungs become the first victim, as the "canopy" of our internal organs (known as such because they occupy the highest position of TCM's five internal organs). The upward reversal of lung energy leads to coughing, and long-term coughing results in deficient lung energy. This would again impair our ability to resist external pathogens. Under such circumstances lung diseases can develop and resist cure. The breakdown of the lungs then may give rise to diseases of the spleen, kidney, heart and other internal organs.

According to *Yellow Emperor's Inner Canon*, people should learn how to give in to Mother Nature, and not try to artificially counteract climatic conditions. In summer we should try to expand our pores so that body heat is emitted, preventing illness. Bathing can also help nourish our lungs. Since the skin and hair are the lungs' screen, bathing can promote the cycle of energy and blood. This will ease the flow of the energy and blood of the lungs and skin, thus moistening and nourishing our lungs.

In addition, often consuming cold drinks in summer can impair the lungs. In summer, according to TCM, it is relatively cold within our body, and our yang is all concentrated in our skin and hair. Upon drinking cold beverages, the additional cold in the body may impair lung function and cause harm. One should not eat many foods that are defined as having "cold" properties in TCM. These include watermelon, bitter gourd, and tomato.

White Food Nourishes Lungs

As we have seen previously, in TCM the five internal organs correspond with the four seasons. In addition, they have relations to certain colors, and the lungs, which correspond with autumn, also relate to the color white.

In autumn the weather is dry, the air temperature declines gradually, and the moisture on the body's surface and the fluid within tend to diminish. Such symptoms as dry skin and flaking of skin often occur. Lungs are in charge of the skin and hair, which function as the channel connecting the lung with the outside. Malnutrition of the skin and hair will surely affect the lungs.

Although the lungs tend to be impaired in autumn, it is actually the best time for nourishing them. This is the season when the energy and function of lungs reach their prime. If we nourish lungs at this opportune time, we can achieve unexpected desirable results.

When it is dry in autumn, eating lung-nourishing food is recommended. *Yellow Emperor's Inner Canon* tells us to moisturize ourselves with various moisture-laden things when it is dry. According to TCM white foods are mostly mild and sweet, with a very good effect of moistening the lungs.

White fungus, an edible fungus, has the best effect of tonifying. It has as many benefits as other moistening foods, such as radix ophiopogon and radix polygonati officinalis, but doesn't have negative qualities, such as being cold or oily. Therefore white fungus is the best food for nourishing yin and moistening the lungs.

Those suffering from a dry nose and lips can eat such

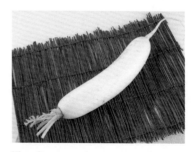

Turnip

foods as snow pear, turnip, sesame, bean curd and soybean milk. In addition, white fungus can tonify the lung and moisten dryness, while walnut can tonify the kidneys and soothe nerves. They produce a stronger curative effect if eaten in autumn.

Recipes to Nourish Lungs

Recipe 1

Ingredients: 5 g white fungus, 10 Chinese dates, 1 snow pear (peeled and sliced), 50 g lotus seeds, rock candy (sugar)

Preparation: Soak white fungus until fully expanded.

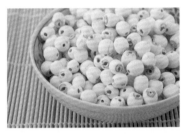

Lotus Seed

Remove base and tear into flakes. Put white fungus, Chinese dates, snow pear and lotus seeds into a pot. Add a moderate amount of water and bring to boil. Then simmer until well-done. Add rock candy to taste, and eat after the rock candy is dissolved.

Note: White fungus, snow pear and lotus seeds serve to moisten the lung, Chinese dates nourish the stomach and spleen, supplement energy, promote production of body fluids, moisten the heart and lungs, and tonify the five internal organs.

Recipe 2

Ingredients: 50 g fresh lily bulb, 30 g honey

Preparation: Brew together and drink.

Recipe 3

Ingredients: 2 pears, 10 g bulbus fritillariae cirrhosae

Preparation: Stew together in water and drink.

Note: Both recipes 2 and 3 have an ideal effect for those who suffer from dry lungs, long-term coughing and chronic bronchitis.

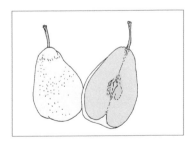

Pear

How to Exercise the Lung Meridian

As we have learned the lungs are the "canopy" of the five internal organs. Therefore frequent rubbing and pressing of the chest area over the lungs can stimulate the Lung Meridian. This promotes the normal operation of the lungs as well as the other internal organs.

The Taiyin Lung Meridian of Hand starts from the upper abdomen, goes downward and contacts the large intestine. Then it returns from the large intestine, goes round the upper mouth of the stomach circularly, and continues upward, passing through the thoracic diaphragm. It contacts the lungs, goes transversely from the trachea, exits the body surface from the armpit and continues along the inside of the upper arm.

On the arm it then moves under the front of the Shaoyin Heart Meridian of Hand and Jueyin Pericardium Meridian of Hand to the inside of the elbow. After passing the radial artery along the inside of the upper arm and lower edge of the radius, it moves forward to the thenar region. It travels along the thenar edge and exits from the inside of the thumb. Another branch separates from behind the wrist, goes toward the inside of the index finger, and meets the Yangming Large Intestine Meridian of Hand.

While the energy and blood of the Lung Meridian reaches its prime at Yin Time (3 a.m. to 5 a.m.), most of us are asleep at

Nourishing the Lung by Breathing Exercises
Breathing exercises, focusing on inhalation and exhalation, can also achieve the effect of nourishing the lung.

During inhalation the tongue presses the palate, the chest expands, the abdomen is drawn in, and energy reaches the lower abdomen. During the exhalation the chest is withdrawn, the abdomen expands, the tongue presses the space between the upper and lower teeth, the lips close slightly, and a hissing sound occurs.

Frequent practice of this method can discharge tainted air and nurse the lungs.

this time. Therefore we normally adjust and nourish our Lung Meridian in the daytime.

Discharge Stagnation: Rub and Knead Yunmen Point

The Yunmen point is located at the center of a pit beside the shoulder clavicle. The simplest way to find it is that you can see

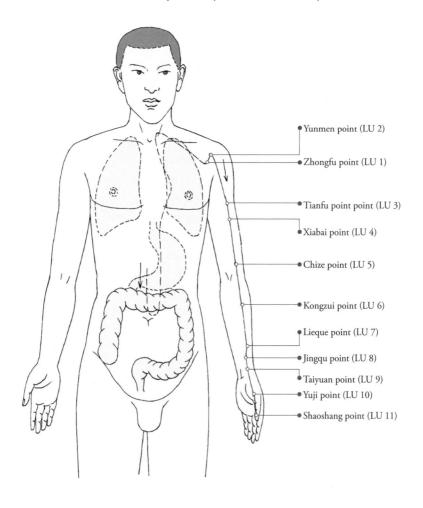

Yunmen point (LU 2)

Zhongfu point (LU 1)

Tianfu point point (LU 3)

Xiabai point (LU 4)

Chize point (LU 5)

Kongzui point (LU 6)

Lieque point (LU 7)

Jingqu point (LU 8)

Taiyuan point (LU 9)

Yuji point (LU 10)

Shaoshang point (LU 11)

Taiyin Lung Meridian of Hand

this pit when you have your hands on hips, with your shoulder exposed.

In irritable people, the vital energy is suffocated in this spot and cannot be let out. As energy goes to the four limbs along the Lung Meridian, crabby people would feel uneasy and hot in their limbs, stifled in the heart and hot in the palms. If the Yunmen point is rubbed and kneaded at this time, affected people may hiccup and the energy continues traveling, going out of their body.

Improve Middle Warmer Energy and Breathing Problems: Rub and Knead Zhongfu Point

The Zhongfu point is located 1 cun below the Yunmen point (described above). If you often feel breathless or feel powerless when defecating, or if you feel flatulent after taking a little food, this indicates that the energy in your spleen and lungs is insufficient. This area is known as the Middle Warmer in TCM. Such symptoms as coughing, asthma, constriction and gasping for breath would occur at the same time. You should rub and knead the Zhongfu point at this time.

Cure Insufficient Lung Energy: Rub and Knead Xiabai Point

If your heartbeat is too fast, or you often feel anxious or suffer from intercostal neuralgia, you can rub and knead this point frequently. The Xiabai point is located on the upper arm where the Lung Meridian passes through, and near the inside of the elbow.

Transfer Energy and Tonify Kidney: Rub and Knead Chize Point

The Chize point is located at the pit beside the elbow. According to *Yellow Emperor's Inner Canon*, the lungs and kidneys belong to gold and water respectively, and gold creates water. Therefore sufficient lung energy can tonify the kidneys. Frequent rubbing and kneading of this point can bring the redundant energy in the Lung Meridian to the Kidney Meridian. "Heat" is also a kind of energy in the body, and it is made from energy and blood. Therefore "heat" cannot be discharged or transferred randomly or without thought.

For example a person may always feel hot and want to eat cool food; however his feet feel icy. This is because his heat has gone upward, leading to the symptom of "upper excess and lower deficiency." Often rubbing and kneading the Chize point can transfer the heat to the Kidney Meridian.

Cure Certain Sore Throats and Fevers: Rub and Knead Kongzui Point

The Kongzui point is located at the cubital crease, 5 cun below the Chize point. It is in charge of all problems related to pores in the human body. In the case of a sore throat caused by a cold, rubbing and kneading this point for 2 to 3 minutes will alleviate or eliminate the soreness. This is effective against fevers without sweating and hemorrhoids as well.

Cure Migraine, Stiff Neck and Prostate Diseases, and Baby Bed-Wetting: Rub and Knead Lieque Point

The Lieque point is located on the lateral edge of the upper arm (aligned with the thumb) and 1.5 cun above the wrist crease. Your index finger touches this point when you cross the thumb-index web of your hands. As one of the four main points of the body, the Lieque point is crucial to curing numerous diseases of the head and neck.

While pressing and rubbing this point, seize the wrist from the direction of the little finger with the other hand. Clasp the back of wrist with the other four fingers, and then press and rub the Lieque point with the tip of the thumb (making sure your thumbnails are not too long). After that exchange your hands to repeat the above action, 3 minutes each time.

Treat Various Heart-Related Problems: Rub and Knead Taiyuan Point

The Taiyuan point is located on the wrist crease, on the side of the thumb. Its function is to regulate and tonify vital energy and to adjust the rhythm of heart.

Some people often cough and gasp very hard, some perspire profusely after undertaking even moderate physical activity, while others feel suffocated, oppressed or inflated in the chest. All of these symptoms can be cured by tonifying or regulating vital energy with this point.

The Taiyuan point is the confluence of all blood vessels, and the heart is in charge of the blood vessels. Therefore the Taiyuan point is apt to cure problems such as heartache, palpitation, arrhythmia and premature beat, among other heart-related conditions.

Treat Heat in Heart, Certain Kinds of Coughing and Insomnia, Pediatric Indigestion: Rub and Knead Yuji Point

The Yuji point is located at a place shaped like a fish belly under the thumb. Pressing this point, the most commonly used point on the Lung Meridian, gives a sense of pain. Since there is a thick layer of muscle at this point, more force should be applied to stimulate the point.

The best way is to rub and knead it with the second joint of the index finger by clenching your fist. After about 3 minutes, exchange your hands and rub for an additional 3 minutes. This method has numerous beneficial effects including curing not only nocturnal coughing, sore throat, hoarse voice, fever, headache, etc., but also preventing mastitis, chest-pain and backache at the time of breathing, swollen fingers and arm pain. It is helpful in treating insomnia caused by stuffiness and agitation as well as pediatric indigestion.

Chapter Four

Mao Time (5 a.m. to 7 a.m.)
Large Intestine Meridian in Its Prime

At Mao Time (5 a.m. to 7 a.m.) the day begins to break and the sun rises slowly. At this time people welcome the rising sun, open their houses, and prepare for the day. Likewise our body is starting a brand-new day. At this time the Yangming Large Intestine Meridian of Hand (Large Intestine Meridian) is in its prime. Punctual defecation can ease the burden of the Large Intestine Meridian and have the healthy effect of lubricating the intestines and expelling toxins.

According to *Yellow Emperor's Inner Canon*, the large intestine concentrates on transporting residues and clearing waste in the human body. After the intake of food, the small intestine digests it, separating and absorbing nutrients, while moving along waste materials at the same time. Transported and transformed by the spleen, these nutrients are spread all over the body to nourish the internal organs. The remains descend to the large intestine, which then absorbs some body fluid found in them. After having been dried in this way, the materials become feces, which are expelled via the anus.

What the large intestine absorbs is only a tiny part of the total fluid in the body. Body fluid maintains the liquid balance of the intestinal canal, acting as a lubricant. People can defecate normally only when the body fluid in the intestinal canal is normal. If the large intestine is so hot that it absorbs too much liquid, the fluid that should have been reserved in the large intestine will be absorbed. The intestinal canal will become dry due to the lack of lubricating body fluid, thus resulting in difficulty in defecation. On the contrary, if the absorption function is too weak and too much liquid remains in the intestinal canal, people can have loose bowel movements.

Warm Water Purges Intestines and Expels Toxins

Daily defecation at a regular time can also promote health. According to TCM there is a relationship of "internal and external coordination" between the large intestine and lungs. When you cannot defecate regularly, you often exert all your strength by holding your breath. Abnormal feces or constipation actually indicate there is a problem with your vital energy, i.e. the energy in your lungs. The lungs are in charge of skin and hair, and therefore constipation may lead to an outbreak of pimples on your face, or a dark and dull complexion. In order to help your Large Intestine Meridian work normally, you must expel waste from your body during this period.

However people often ignore this. Some defecate at an improper time, while others cannot defecate easily. In the former case, it is best to make adjustments to conform to the laws of nature; because the large intestine works at Mao Time, this is the most appropriate time to go to the toilet. In the case of the latter, one must try to discover the causes. If pain or burning is experienced at the time of defecation, one should avoid or eat less spicy food. If there is pain in the stomach or abdomen, and one cannot defecate at all, this indicates that the daily diet is too oily and lacks roughage. The feces accumulated in the large intestine have become a pathogenic factor.

The process of treating constipation starts with a glass of warm water. Drinking this on an empty stomach in the early morning can purge your intestines and stomach, promote the clearance of toxins, facilitate defecation and provide refreshment.

Some people add salt to their water, believing this can promote health. However the opposite is true. During overnight sleep, such activities as breathing, perspiration and urination still go on. These consume a lot of water, yet no water is taken in during sleep. Therefore people usually have the highest blood pressure in the early morning. If they drink lightly salted water at this time, their blood may possibly become more concentrated. In particular, patients with cardiovascular disease usually have very viscose blood when they get up, and salt water would further exacerbate this condition.

If you dislike the neutral or plain taste of water, you can add some honey to it. Honey, which has the function of relaxing bowels, is nutritious and can replenish in a timely manner the vital energy you have consumed overnight. Therefore honey is beneficial for one's health.

Tonifying Spleen and Kidneys Cures Morning Diarrhea

According to TCM, morning diarrhea is attributed to insufficient vital yang energy in the spleen and kidneys. Therefore promoting the yang energy in these organs can cure morning diarrhea. How can we do this? Massaging the Zusanli point, an acupoint of the Yangming Stomach Meridian of Foot, every day can cure all deficiency syndromes. Therefore we can use this method to cure the deficiency of yang in the spleen and kidneys.

Frequently stimulating the Zusanli point can reinforce the kidneys, boost essence, warm the spleen, increase yang, and promote longevity. The Zusanli point is located by moving the distance spanned by four transverse fingers under the outer knee depression, on the edge of the shin bone. In other words if you cover your kneecap with your palm, fingers facing downward,

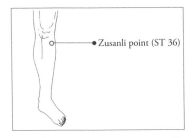

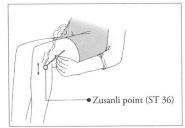

Practicing massage, acupuncture and/ or moxibustion over the Zusanli point can reinforce the kidney, boost essence, warm the spleen and increase yang.

Moxibustion over the Zusanli point is particularly effective in curing deficiency of yang in the spleen and kidneys.

then the tip of your middle finger will be exactly located at this acupoint.

You can press and knead this point with your thumb for about five minutes, preferably using enough strength to produce a sense of soreness and heat.

You can also use the method of moxibustion, igniting a moxa stick and slowly moving it up and down along your Zusanli point, preferably making your skin slightly hot without burning it. You can practice this two to three times a week for 15 to 20 minutes a time. If you persist in practicing this for one to two months, you can cure the deficiency of yang in your spleen and kidneys.

Food Therapy

In addition to massaging the Zusanli point, you can also use food therapy, adding to your diet more foods classified as warm in TCM (such as mutton soup with Angelica sinensis, the recipe for which follows). According to the classical text *Synopsis of Golden Chamber*, Angelica sinensis has the function of nourishing and tonifying blood. Ginger can warm the spleen and stomach, dispel cold, induce sweat and dispel toxins. Mutton is also warm-natured, and can warm the spleen and stomach, and tonify deficiencies. Therefore mutton can have a good effect on people with deficient vital energy and blood and insufficient yang energy.

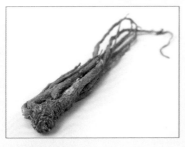

Recipe of Mutton Soup with Angelica Sinensis
Ingredients: 3–5 g Angelica sinensis, 30 g ginger, 500 g mutton.

Preparation: Place the mutton in a pot of boiling water, blanch, and wash the mutton clean. Remove the fascia and cut the mutton into pieces. Cut the ginger into slices. Place the Angelica sinensis, mutton and sliced ginger into the pot, and add a suitable amount of clear water, cooking wine and salt. Cook on high heat until the water boils. Then simmer for 2 hours. Finally add MSG to taste and sprinkle with some chopped green onion. Eat the mutton as well as the soup.

Angelica Sinensis

However the food mentioned above is not suitable for people who tend to get inflamed, or have a cold accompanied with a fever, or have a sore throat.

Proper Dining Keeps Intestinal Canal Healthy

Dining properly encompasses several factors: in addition to eating at the right time, one must also pay attention to achieving balance, controlling the ratio between staples and non-staples, not eating highly-processed foods, and fully chewing the food.

Nowadays some people, especially some girls influenced by beauty images, choose not to eat staple foods so as to maintain their slim figures. This habit tends to cause diseases. According to experts in this area, long-term avoidance of staple foods and the intake of too much fat result in the frequent occurrence of colorectal cancer. Insufficient intake of staple foods gives rise to the lack of protein, minerals, vitamins and other useful substances in the body, as well as the decline of the body's immunity.

As far as we know, more than 90% of immune organs in the

human body are distributed in the intestinal canal; the breakdown of our immune system would result in the multiplication of problems with our intestinal canal. Furthermore not eating staple foods would give rise to serious

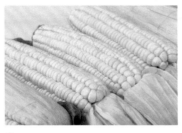
Corn

lack of dietary fiber thus leading to constipation, which over the long term can trigger colorectal cancer.

Some people eat only finely-processed rice or flour as their staple food, which is a bad habit. This results in the lack of dietary fiber in the body, which is detrimental to the health of the large intestine. More and more people have been suffering from colorectal cancer in recent years, which can be attributed to the intake of insufficient dietary fiber.

In addition to flour and rice, we should eat a moderate amount of corn, millet, purple rice, sorghum, oat, buckwheat, wheat bran, soybean, green bean, red bean and mung bean, so as to increase the coarse fiber in our body, promote movement of the intestinal canal, and boost the digestion and absorption of nutritious food. Experts believe that some rhizomatic foods also contain rich dietary fiber and a lot of vitamins. Therefore this kind of food (e.g. potato, sweet potato and taro) has a strong function of protecting the abdomen, relaxing the bowels and enhancing immunity, and can also be eaten as a staple food.

However the intake of too much coarse grain is inadvisable, and should only comprise part of one's diet. In particular, elderly people are advised not to take in too much coarse grain, and it should preferably account for one-third of their total staple foods.

We should not only pay attention to balance in our diet, but also to the speed of dining. Eating too rapidly harms the intestine. Directly swallowing food into the intestine and stomach without fully chewing adds burden to these organs. This not only prevents food from being fully digested and absorbed, but also brings about many consequences to health in the long run, e.g. intestinal diseases, obesity, malnutrition, memory loss and slow reaction.

Therefore we must develop good dining habits in our daily life. In review, we must eat staple foods every day, maintaining the right balance between processed and coarse grain. Only in this way can we strive to nip large intestine diseases in the bud, and maintain intestinal health.

Relax Bowels and Prevent Hemorrhoids

Problems with the large intestine usually lead to constipation, which can also produce many complications, such as hemorrhoids. Hemorrhoids are quite common, but how do they come into being?

Hemorrhoids occur at the end of large intestine, i.e. anus, a place where there are many blood vessels. It is hard for the blood in some of these vessels to flow back to the liver. Therefore such circumstances as uneven blood flow and blood stasis tend to occur in these parts. In particular at the time of defecation, people experience exertion, and the pressure in the abdomen increases at this time. Therefore a lot of blood cannot flow back after flowing to the anus and intestine. Blood stasis becomes more serious at the location of the anus. Patients with constipation have difficulty in defecation. When they exert force to try to relieve this condition, the anus bears a high pressure, and the blood vessels there accumulate clots, thus giving rise to phlebangioma, i.e. hemorrhoids. These can be quite painful.

Long-term hematochezia (rectal bleeding) also leads to iron-deficiency anemia. Although this symptom caused by hemorrhoids is not obvious in the early period, too much blood is lost as time goes on, and patients develop such symptoms as facial pallor, lassitude, loss of appetite, palpitation, edema, fidgetiness and unstable mood. Therefore patients with hemorrhoids are advised to see a doctor as soon as these symptoms occur, in case the symptoms should become serious.

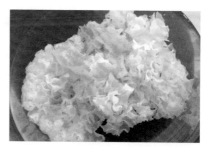

White Fungus

The occurrence of hemorrhoids is closely related to the large intestine. In particular, constipation must be cured as soon as possible, because it can promote the occurrence of hemorrhoids. Diet is an important factor in preventing hemorrhoids, as well as alleviating symptoms

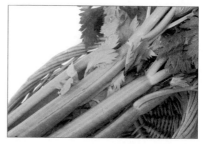

Celery

and reducing recurrence. One should eat more food that can relax the bowels, such as white fungus, lily bulb, Chinese leek, wild rice shoots, celery, spinach, yogurt, honey, sesame, pine nut, walnut and other foods containing rich cellulose, which can promote movement of the intestines and stomach, and relax the bowels.

Patients with hemorrhoids should be sure to avoid or consume less spicy or pungent food, e.g. pepper, mustard, ginger, liquor, yellow rice wine, garlic and onion, because they stimulate the mucosa skin of the rectum and anus, and intensify such symptoms as the hemorrhage and prolapse of hemorrhoids.

It is also advised that hemorrhoid sufferers should not eat too much food. Their feces can then become dry enough to make defecation difficult, thus intensifying the symptoms of hemorrhoids and increasing the difficulty of treatment. In addition, patients should do more physical exercise, promote their blood circulation, develop a habit of timely defecation, and control the time of defecation, which will promote treatment and recovery.

Recommended Foods for Preventing Hemorrhoids

1. Black sesame has the function of relaxing the bowels, and alleviating the hemorrhage and prolapse of hemorrhoids.

2. Honey can tonify and relax the bowels.

3. Red beans can cure the hemorrhage and swelling of hemorrhoids if decocted together with Angelica sinensis. It is also excellent in preventing and curing hemorrhoids when made into a porridge alone or together with rice.

4. Flos sophorae, which can cool the blood, stop bleeding and remove hemorrhoids, can be made into a cold dish or dumplings, or taken as a tea.

5. Walnuts can relax the bowels, tonify deficiency, and alleviate such symptoms as the hemorrhage and prolapse of hemorrhoids.

6. Bamboo shoots, containing abundant cellulose, help in relaxing the bowels.

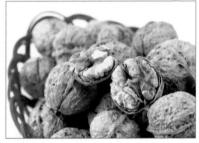

Walnut

How to Exercise the Large Intestine Meridian

Abbreviated as the Large Intestine Meridian, the full name of this meridian is the Yangming Large Intestine Meridian of Hand. It starts at the Shangyang point and ends at the Yingxiang point, with 20 points located on its left and right respectively. It connects such parts as the mouth, teeth, nose, lung, large intestine and arm. You can exercise your Large Intestine Meridian frequently by patting the meridian and by rubbing and kneading the Hegu point. Often patting this meridian can cure toothache, sore throat, numb upper limbs, stomachache, borborygmus, constipation, diarrhea and other symptoms.

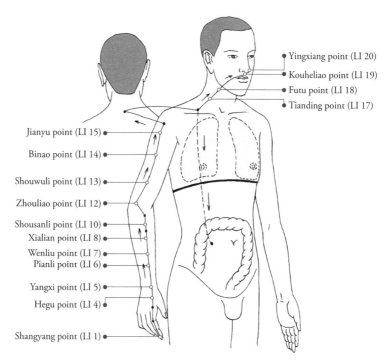

Yingxiang point (LI 20)
Kouheliao point (LI 19)
Futu point (LI 18)
Tianding point (LI 17)

Jianyu point (LI 15)

Binao point (LI 14)

Shouwuli point (LI 13)

Zhouliao point (LI 12)

Shousanli point (LI 10)
Xialian point (LI 8)
Wenliu point (LI 7)
Pianli point (LI 6)

Yangxi point (LI 5)
Hegu point (LI 4)

Shangyang point (LI 1)

Yangming Large Intestine Meridian of Hand

Tapping the Large Intestine Meridian

Frequently tapping the Large Intestine Meridian can deal with a number of symptoms including toothache, sore throat, numb arms, stomachache, borborygmus, constipation and diarrhea.

Clench your right hand lightly into a hollow fist, bend your arm, and reach across to the left. Let your left hand fall naturally at your side. Begin to tap it upward with your right hand, moving from the wrist, across the elbow and to the shoulder, for a total of six minutes. Then repeat on the other side, patting your right arm with your left hand. Do not exert too much force during tapping.

If you practice this once a day, you will not only invigorate the vital energy and blood in your Large Intestine Meridian and

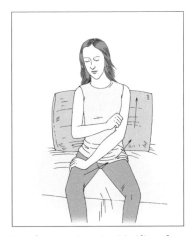

Tap the Large Intestine Meridian often to alleviate some symptoms.

keep it functioning smoothly, but also reduce the possibility of constipation and diarrhea. In addition, tapping it often can relieve fatigue and pain in your arms, alleviate arm strain, and relax yourself both physically and mentally.

Office workers who sit at a computer for a whole day, and drivers who operate vehicles all day may feel tingling, numb and a lack of strength in their arms, or even feel pain. Frequently tapping the Large Intestine Meridian can not only alleviate these symptoms very well, but also allow people to better dedicate themselves to work.

Rub and Knead Hegu Point

The Large Intestine Meridian has a very noticeable acupoint on the hand: the Hegu point. It is found between the bones of the thumb and first finger, on the back of the hand, and can be reached with the thumb tip of the opposite hand.

According to collateral and meridian theory, along with practical proof, massaging the Hegu point can alleviate or eliminate diseases of the tissues and organs passed through circularly by the Large Intestine Meridian (to which the Hegu point belongs), thus ensuring health. Since the Large Intestine Meridian starts from the hand and runs through the head, massaging the Hegu point can help alleviate or cure all head and face diseases, e.g. headache, fever, thirst, nosebleed, swelling neck, throat disease and other diseases of the five sense organs.

Massaging first one hand and then the other, press down on the Hegu point with the bent thumb of the other hand, once every other second, i.e. about 30 times a minute. It is important to exert a relatively strong force while pressing this point, working until tingling, numbness and swelling actually occur to the point.

This method can not only prevent and cure diseases of the eyes, ears, nose, mouth and throat (e.g. swelling and sore throat, coldness, nasal obstruction, cough and asthma) but also produce a good curative effect for such problems as constipation, diarrhea and vomiting. Please note that it is preferable for the Large Intestine Meridian to be maintained and exercised in the time period from 5 to 7 a.m., because the vital energy and blood of the Large Intestine Meridian are at their prime at this time.

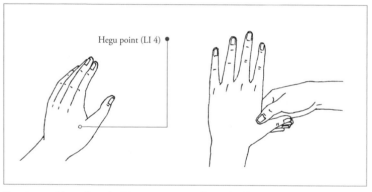

Hegu point (LI 4)

Pressing and kneading the Hegu point can effectively alleviate and cure many ailments, including headache, fever, thirst, nosebleed, throat problems, constipation, diarrhea and vomiting.

Chapter Five

Chen Time (7 a.m. to 9 a.m.)
Stomach Meridian in Its Prime

At Chen Time (7 a.m. to 9 a.m.) the sun has already risen, and with warm sunshine illuminating the earth, the body feels comfortable. However after being consumed as fuel overnight, the food in our stomach has been digested completely. Therefore the first thing we should do at Chen Time is to eat so as to replenish energy. Chen Time is exactly when the Yangming Stomach Meridian of Foot (Stomach Meridian) is in its prime. Food, after having been absorbed and digested by the stomach, can soon be turned into the energy needed by the body. This is why we feel energetic immediately after breakfast.

According to *Yellow Emperor's Inner Canon*, the stomach is an organ that stores food, the source of nutrition for the activity of our internal organs, and the center that we rely on for survival. Due to the accelerating pace of life, many people have developed a bad habit of skipping breakfast in order to save time or trouble. In addition, some people, particularly girls, feel that breakfast will make them fat, and therefore avoid it.

This is a misunderstanding, and one should not worry about eating a lot of food at Chen Time. The spleen and kidneys can digest and absorb food efficiently at this time, and the Stomach Meridian can completely digest the food we have taken in. It will transform the food into the energy needed by our body (instead of storing it as fat), transporting it all over the body to support the internal organs.

Therefore we should eat enough breakfast at Chen Time, following the natural rhythm of the body; otherwise the Stomach Meridian will have nothing to do but secrete too much gastric acid. This may lead to disorders of the digestion system, causing such problems as gastric ulcer, gastritis and duodenitis in the long run. In addition to gastric diseases, skipping breakfast completely or not eating enough may directly result in cardiocerebrovascular diseases as well as hepatic and biliary diseases.

It is clear that not eating a proper breakfast is harmful, and it is important to eat it at the right time. In order to maintain health and beauty, breakfast is key.

Optimize Nutrition through Food Choices

Since breakfast is vital, how and what should we eat? The answer is simple: We should eat what our stomach likes and absorbs readily. For example warm food won't cause discomfort to the stomach, and can be absorbed by the stomach very well before being transformed into the energy needed by the body. In addition, combining foods in different ways affects taste and nutritional value.

A food deserving particular mention here is porridge. If rice is stewed with a temperature higher than 60 degrees, gelatinization occurs. Therefore rice porridge (also known as congee) can be digested easily without making the stomach uncomfortable. Rice porridge plus pickled vegetables is a nutritious, appetizing and ideal breakfast, and is quite common as a traditional breakfast in China.

You can also add some ingredients into the bland porridge to boost taste and nutrition. For example Chinese dates can replenish

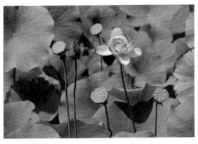

Lotus Leaves

the blood and invigorate the spleen, pearl barleys can enhance and moisten the skin, angelica sinensis can replenish vitality and nourish the blood, and lotus leaves can clear away heart-heat and relieve summer heat.

In addition to using various condiments, porridge can be eaten together with some other foods, e.g. tasty vegetables, poached eggs, lean meat or fruit. Porridge not only allays hunger, but is also an ideal form of food therapy. Furthermore porridge has such efficacies as caring for the intestines and stomach, whetting appetite, preventing constipation and colds, and helping to prolong life. Therefore porridge is an optimal choice for the early morning.

Do not eat overly cold food as your breakfast, such as iced fruit juices or even cold water; otherwise stomach-cold occurs. The Stomach Meridian works at Chen Time, when yang energy reaches its peak, and energy and blood are plentiful. These will stagnate when cooled. Food that is too cold results in uneven energy and blood of the Stomach Meridian, and may give rise to gastric spasm or gastric discomfort. In the long run, the function of the intestines and stomach will decline, thus bringing about malnutrition, a withered and sallow complexion, and lassitude and emaciation.

In terms of traditional Chinese medicine, in normal cases the stomach secretes mucus to protect the stomach wall, as well as digestive juice and gastric acid to promote digestion. So-called "stomach-cold" is caused by insufficient energy, which refers to low gastric function and insufficient elasticity of the gastric muscle. This affects the peristalsis of the stomach and the supply of secretions. Insufficient digestive juice and gastric acid can lead to a sluggish stomach, loss of appetite, and an all-day feeling of abdominal distention or even vomiting. The above-mentioned symptoms may be attributed to having eaten too much cold food.

Maintain Beauty by Tapping Stomach Meridian

One key to beauty is to maintain an unblocked Stomach Meridian and plentiful energy and blood. In order to enhance the complexion, frequently tapping the Stomach Meridian is advised.

Beauty is closely related to the Stomach Meridian. As is widely known, maintaining an optimal internal condition is more important than external treatment for promoting beauty. This includes taking care of the Yangming Stomach Meridian of Foot. The functions of the stomach and spleen, and the free flow of the Stomach Meridian, ensure sufficient energy and blood in the internal organs. This will help to make women's faces rosy, lustrous and glowing, as energy and vitality coming from within is the most important factor in beauty. "A face like a peach blossom" was often used in ancient China to refer to a beautiful girl. This phrase indicates the woman has an unblocked Stomach Meridian, and sufficient energy and blood, creating a glowing face and healthy body.

The Stomach Meridian starts from the nose, joins at the root of the nose, goes downward along the outside of the nose, enters the upper-teeth socket, goes out of the mouth and circles the lips. It then continues downward and joins at the mentolabial sulcus and moves along both sides to the angle of the mandible. Proceeding upward, it passes the front of the ear and zygoma, and advances along the hairline to the center of the forehead and cranium. Its externally-moving trunk goes down from the supraclavicular fossa, passes such acupoints as the Ruzhong point, descends along both sides of the navel,

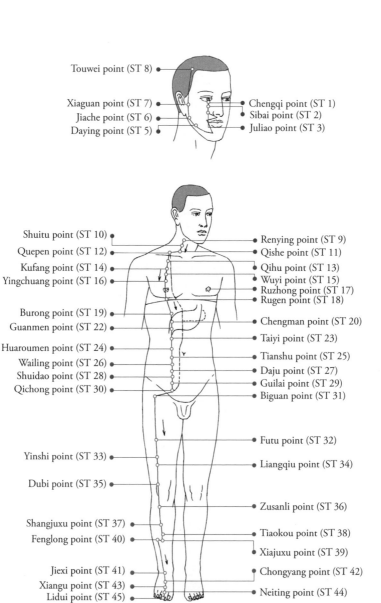

Touwei point (ST 8)

Xiaguan point (ST 7)
Jiache point (ST 6)
Daying point (ST 5)

Chengqi point (ST 1)
Sibai point (ST 2)
Juliao point (ST 3)

Shuitu point (ST 10)
Quepen point (ST 12)
Kufang point (ST 14)
Yingchuang point (ST 16)

Renying point (ST 9)
Qishe point (ST 11)
Qihu point (ST 13)
Wuyi point (ST 15)
Ruzhong point (ST 17)
Rugen point (ST 18)

Burong point (ST 19)
Guanmen point (ST 22)

Chengman point (ST 20)
Taiyi point (ST 23)

Huaroumen point (ST 24)
Wailing point (ST 26)
Shuidao point (ST 28)
Qichong point (ST 30)

Tianshu point (ST 25)
Daju point (ST 27)
Guilai point (ST 29)
Biguan point (ST 31)

Futu point (ST 32)

Yinshi point (ST 33)

Liangqiu point (ST 34)

Dubi point (ST 35)

Zusanli point (ST 36)

Shangjuxu point (ST 37)
Fenglong point (ST 40)

Tiaokou point (ST 38)
Xiajuxu point (ST 39)

Jiexi point (ST 41)
Xiangu point (ST 43)
Lidui point (ST 45)

Chongyang point (ST 42)
Neiting point (ST 44)

Yangming Stomach Meridian of Foot

and enters the common channel where the energy of different meridians comes together.

The Stomach Meridian has four sub-meridians. The first sub-meridian starts from the front of the angle of the mandible, goes past the carotid artery and along the throat, enters the supraclavicular fossa, passes the diaphragm, and then becomes part of the stomach and links itself with spleen. The second sub-meridian starts from the stomach, goes along the inside of the abdomen, and joins the externally-moving trunk at the artery of the groin. It then goes downward, passes the front of the hip joint, and moves along the outside of the leg. Finally it goes onto the dorsum of the feet, enters the interior crevice of the middle toe, and exits at the end of the second toe. The third sub-meridian separates three cun below the knee, goes downward, enters the exterior crevice of the middle toe, and goes out at the end of the middle toe. The fourth sub-meridian separates from the dorsum of the feet, enters the crevice of the hallux toe, goes out at the end of this toe, and connects with the Taiyin Spleen Meridian of Foot.

As seen in the illustration, the Stomach Meridian runs through the entire body from the head to feet. As long as we ensure its smooth operation, our energy and blood will remain sufficient, keeping us radiant with good health.

How can one condition the Stomach Meridian? There is a simple way, which does not require much expense or time. You need only to frequently tap the Yangming Stomach Meridian of Foot whenever you have a little spare time. From the face, press downward gently with all ten fingers. Tap the neck gently with the palm, and tap the section running from the neck to the leg with a fist. Increase force gradually, but never apply an extremely strong force. Be sure to temper your force depending on the bearing capacity of our body.

Quench Liver Fire to Protect and Nourish Spleen and Stomach

As we have learned earlier, according to *Yellow Emperor's Inner Canon*, anger can hurt the liver, and too much liver fire affects the spleen and stomach. This can lead to loss of appetite and low spirits. While liver fire is affected by mood, food may also bring about too much liver-heat.

The spleen, stomach and liver are all digestive organs, and they are as closely related as brothers. Only when they coexist harmoniously and cooperate with each other can food be digested, absorbed and metabolized normally.

The major function of the stomach is storing and absorbing food, and the liver is a filtering screen in the digestive system. All food in the stomach is filtered by the liver, so that toxins in the food can be removed. Some fried, spicy or pickled food may contain toxins, as may some food treated with chemical pesticide or processed with additives, and even some chemically synthesized drugs. The toxins can be discharged only after having been processed by the liver, so as to minimize their harm to the body. If too many hazardous substances are taken into the stomach, the liver is forced to work beyond its capacity, which it is unable to sustain in the long run. This gives rise to liver hyperemia and liver fire.

The most direct reactions to too much liver-heat include lassitude, loss of appetite, and even dizziness, giddiness, agitation, irritability, insomnia, impotence and premature ejaculation. Therefore too much liver-heat must be treated seriously.

Quenching liver-heat should begin from dietary conditioning. Porridge in the early morning, with a mild nature and a sweet taste, is recommended. Adding Chinese dates into the porridge can invigorate the spleen, nourish the stomach and protect the liver. In addition, we should try to eat little or no dried, pickled or irritating food, and should also refrain from eating chemically-processed food, e.g. food with additives. Vegetables and fruits that contain chemical pesticides should be thoroughly cleaned before being eaten.

In addition to dietary conditioning, massaging acupoints is recommended, as according to TCM, dredging our meridians promotes blood circulation and has curative effects. In addition to massaging the face, we can tap our legs and massage the Yanglingquan point, which is also a key means of quenching our liver-heat. This point is located below the knee and at the depression in front of the fibula capitulum, outside the shin. Press it with the thumb with due force and massage for three minutes. Be consistent and continue with your practice daily. This method can produce a strong effect of quenching liver-heat.

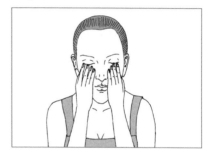

Massaging the Face
Kneading the face with both hands clears a section of the Stomach Meridian running through the face.

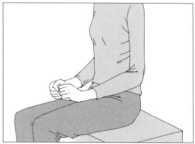

Tapping the Leg
This can dredge the Stomach Meridian and maintain normal circulation of energy and blood.

Yanglingquan Point
Pressing this point with the thumb, and massaging it persistently can effectively quench liver-heat.

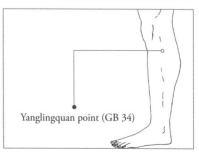

Yanglingquan point (GB 34)

Increase Longevity by Pressing and Kneading Zusanli Point

According to an old Chinese saying, around the age of 30, people are in a golden period, gradually moving toward maturity and beginning to develop their career by working hard. From a physiological perspective, function matures gradually before the age of 30, and reaches its peak at 30. However the age of 30 also indicates the beginning of the move toward mental and physical deterioration. One of the manifestations is that yangming energy in the Yangming Stomach Meridian of Foot is also beginning to decline, with diseases approaching silently. Restraining the "dry gold" energy of yangming can naturally slow down aging.

Yellow Emperor's Inner Canon notes that massaging and using acupuncture at the Zusanli point can slow down aging and enhance longevity. The Zusanli point is located three cun below the outer knee socket, and a horizontal finger-width outside the front ridge of the shin bone. In order to live a longer and healthier life, we should often apply moxibustion to this point.

For best results, place the moxa directly on the chosen acupoint and ignite it; when the moxa column is about to burn out and you feel very hot, keep it on the acupoint until the acupoint is scalded. Keep dry the portion of the skin that is burnt and begins to produce pus. Although this may sound unpleasant, the practice has a basis in medical theory.

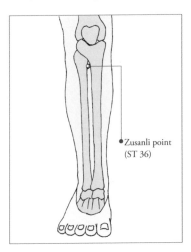

Zusanli point
(ST 36)

Location of Zusanli Point

Zusanli is a point at which the Yangming Stomach Meridian of Foot comes together. After arriving from the ends of the four limbs, the meridian energy reaches its peak and joins the

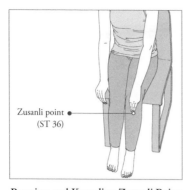

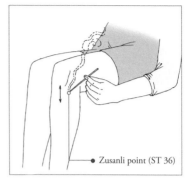

Zusanli point
(ST 36)

Zusanli point (ST 36)

Pressing and Kneading Zusanli Point

One method is to sit with shins stretched forward, maintaining an angle of 120° between the legs and stool, and press and knead with the index finger and middle finger on the Zusanli point.

Moxibustion at Zusanli Point

Practicing moxibustion at this acupoint can deliver heat through to the inside of the body, eliminate some dry yang energy and help in getting rid of diseases.

"sea" just like a stream. Moxibustion can deliver heat to the inside of body through this acupoint, so as to eliminate some dry and yang energy, which will help in getting rid of diseases. Nowadays in order to avoid scalding, people often adopt a relatively mild method of partition-based moxibustion. Such objects as ginger slices are stacked between the moxa stick and the skin. Although this method achieves a weaker effect than the above-mentioned method, repeating it several times can also achieve the same results.

In addition to moxibustion, massaging the Zusanli point can promote healthcare and longevity. Sit on a stool with fingers folded, then press and place the fingers on the outside of the shin. Place the tip of the thumb at the Zusanli point and press. Practice the point-and-press action, pressing and releasing for 36 repetitions; do this to both sides in turn. Or sit on the stool with shin stretched forward, maintaining an angle of 120° between the legs and stool. Press and place the index finger on the Zusanli point, with the middle finger on top of the index finger to add pressure. Press and knead the point with the force of both fingers, continuing for one minute, starting with the right leg and then massaging the left leg. If you persist in practicing this every day, you will achieve a desirable effect.

It is best to practice moxibustion and massage of the Zusanli point at Chen Time (7 to 9 a.m.). At this time, energy and blood flow past the Stomach Meridian, the blood and energy in the stomach are sufficient, and the activity of the meridian reaches its peak. Therefore practicing moxibustion and massage at this time achieves better effect with less effort. If one does not have time to do moxibustion in the early morning, massaging the acupoint during one's commute to work is advised. In the case of inconvenience, the time of practice can also be adjusted slightly.

Prevent Pimples by Overcoming Stomach-Cold

Pimples, also called acne, are a common skin problem. In addition to children, about 50% to 70% of people experience the problem to different extents, with prevalence during the adolescent period. Pimples mostly appear on the face, chest, back and shoulders, with the most common location being the face. They are usually small conical red lumps, with some of them having black heads or white spots. Some are accompanied by aches or itching.

What are the causes of this condition? If analyzed from the perspective of traditional Chinese medicine, a pimple is mostly a skin inflammation caused by too much heat accumulated in body, which relates to stomach-cold.

The Stomach Meridian passes through many of the parts where pimples tend to form, such as the face, chest, back, shoulders and particularly the nose and lips. The abnormality of the Stomach Meridian is often reflected through these parts. Pimples can also reflect problems with the function of the stomach and intestines, i.e. the problem of stomach-cold.

There are many causes of stomach-cold, for example drinking cold beverages too often. Nowadays there are many varieties of cold drinks, and many people are fond of them, drinking them in hot summer and even in cold winter. This tends to bring about stomach-cold.

In general our internal temperature is constant. Once invaded by cold, the body instinctively emits heat to resist the cold. This kind of heat is called "dry heat." This is just like a siege: one party attempts to enter through a violent attack, while the other party tries to guard the city wall and drive away the enemy. In this case one party attacks with coldness, while the other guards with heat. As a result, although the "city wall" is successfully guarded, the dry heat is so vigorous that it is emitted continuously to the outside. The skin becomes its outlet, resulting in acne.

Why are pimples more common among young people, instead of middle-aged or older people? This is because young people have so much energy and blood that they leap up and down in the body. When there is cold air in the stomach, the dry yang air in the body rapidly rises upward together with the cold air, searching everywhere for places to break through to the surface. Face skin becomes the best channel, thus giving rise to pimples.

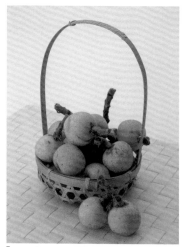

Long-term depression and tension also bring about stomach-cold and pimples on the face. This is why some people exhibit acne on their face beyond adolescence. Extremely high pressure in daily work and life, and heavy mental burden, easily result in

Loquat

loss of appetite and the decline of food digestion and absorption. In the long run, stomach-cold occurs. As we have seen, in order to resist the cold, the dry heat in the body rises upward along with the cold and exits the body, with the face skin as an outlet. As a result, pimples occur on the facial skin.

Since stomach-cold can bring about acne, how should we prevent and cure this condition? One key is to adjust dining habits: drink fewer cold beverages, eat more vegetables and fruits containing a rich amount of fiber (for example, carrot, tomato and sweet potatos), and often drink water. Young people should learn how to adjust and relax themselves, alternate work with rest, maintain an optimistic attitude, ensure eight hours of sleep every day, and refrain from staying up late. People who suffer from indigestion should develop a habit of timely defecation and drink a glass of water after getting up every morning. They should also drink a glass of milk while having breakfast, which can assist coliform in generating lactic acid and promote movement of the intestines. It is also recommended to keep one's face clean every day and take necessary protective measures such as sunscreen.

Cure Halitosis by Eliminating Stomach Heat

Many people have faced an awkward situation brought about by halitosis, or bad breath. Not only do they feel uncomfortable, but it also makes others reluctant to interact with them. Although halitosis is not a lethal disease, we cannot ignore it. It can not only prevent sufferers from associating with others, but also do some psychological harm and make them self-contemptuous and reticent.

In terms of TCM, halitosis is closely related to stomach heat. People suffering from stomach heat usually exhibit symptoms such as constipation, stomachache, indigestion and agitation. So much food is accumulated that the retention of contents occurs, and when the contents cannot be evacuated, it ferments abnormally and produces smells. These smells flow back to the mouth, giving rise to halitosis.

How can we cure halitosis once and for all? It is not enough to only keep our mouths clean every day, but we must also cure it radically. Stomach heat must be eliminated before curing halitosis. Some important acupoints can help in this process: Laogong and Neiting. All these acupoints have the efficacy of eliminating stomach heat and curing halitosis. The frequent massaging of these acupoints can refresh your breath slowly.

The Neiting point is located between the second and third toe. Massaging this acupoint can eliminate stomach-heat. Laogong is an important acupoint on the palm, located exactly at the palm's center, between the second and third metacarpal bones. When making a fist by bending the fingers, the place to which the tip of the middle finger points is the Laogong point. As an important acupoint on the Jueyin Pericardium Meridian of Hand, Laogong has a very strong ability of clearing heat and fire. Therefore this point is often used clinically to treat aphtha and halitosis caused by body-heat or internal heat, with a very obvious effect.

Massaging of the Laogong and Neiting points can help to cure halitosis. For best results, rub and knead each acupoint with the thumb for five minutes, two to three times a day according to symptoms. If you persist in doing so for a week, the symptoms should be relieved very well.

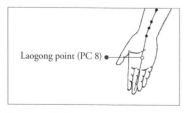
Laogong point (PC 8) •

Laogong Point

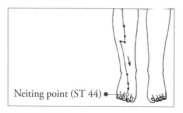
Neiting point (ST 44) •

Neiting Point

Chapter Six

Si Time (9 a.m. to 11 a.m.)
Spleen Meridian in Its Prime

After the breakfast food enters the stomach at Chen Time, the spleen becomes busy at Si Time (9 a.m. to 11 a.m.). We must pay attention to protecting and nourishing the spleen in order to live a longer and healthier life, and it is most effective to care for it at Si Time.

The spleen and stomach are described in *Yellow Emperor's Inner Canon* as the "barn official," a very important administrator in ancient China in charge of the entry and exit of local grains. Just like the barn official, our spleen and stomach are responsible for taking in food, transforming it after due digestion and absorption, and delivering nutrition to all our tissues and organs. According to TCM the spleen is "the foundation of acquired constitution and the source of the generation and transformation of vital energy and blood." This means it has an important role on individual characteristics and health.

Deficiency of spleen energy results in the malfunction of digesting, absorbing and delivering nutritional substances. If organs cannot obtain sufficient energy, a series of pathological changes will occur related to the physiological malfunction of spleen, e.g. anorexia, low spirits, dizziness, abdominal distension, diarrhea and emaciation, and even prolapse of the anus and visceroptosis.

In addition, the spleen is in charge of blood. According to the record of *Synopsis of Golden Chamber*, spleen energy has a function of astringent therapy over blood, ensuring that blood moves in vessels without overflowing, thus preventing hemorrhage. Only when the spleen works normally can the blood circulate in the body. If the spleen energy is so weak that it cannot regulate the function of blood, then such symptoms as hematuria, hematochezia, subcutaneous hemorrhage, metrorrhagia and metrostaxis may occur.

Therefore we must try to regulate and nurture our spleen every day. Since the spleen has an outlet at the mouth, we can also judge whether the spleen is insufficient by observing the tongue. If the tongue is light-colored and there is a trace of being bitten by teeth at the edge, then there is probably a problem with the spleen.

The insufficiency of the spleen is mostly caused by dietary disorder, labor-rest imbalance and weakness due to chronic diseases. Problems with the spleen can be caused if our daily diet is so uniform that the body cannot absorb enough nutrition. In addition, if one works excessively without taking enough rest, if sedentary people or chronic bedridden patients do not take enough physical exercise, or if the muscles are not exercised properly, then the spleen would of course refuse to work hard, as the spleen is in charge of all muscles.

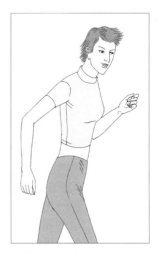

As one of TCM's five internal organs, the spleen is vital for the human body. Many common ailments originate from problems with the spleen, e.g. diabetes, obesity and drooling or excess saliva production.

Sufficient physical exercise protects spleen.

Prevent Diabetes by Caring for Spleen Meridian

In recent years the number of diabetes patients has been growing gradually, and increasing numbers of younger people, and even some children, have been contracting diabetes. Moreover it is quite difficult to radically cure diabetes at the present medical level. Diabetes has become a widespread epidemic.

There are many causes of diabetes, including irregular diet, eating and drinking too much, eating too much fatty food, excessive drinking and depression. The preceding chapter also mentioned a connection of diabetes with the Stomach Meridian. In fact if the operation of the Spleen Meridian is not smooth it can also result in diabetes. The most common expressions of diabetes include over-eating, drinking too much or excessive thirst, excessive urination and gradual emaciation.

From the perspective of traditional Chinese medicine, diabetes is caused by the liver and spleen's heat transformation against cold. The liver and spleen become so hot that the lungs are burned, thus giving rise to lung dryness. This leads to extreme thirst, when one still feels thirsty no matter how much water one drinks.

If this heat cannot be held back in time, it continues to go downward to the stomach, giving rise to stomach dryness as well. At this moment, diabetes patients feel compelled to eat a great deal because the digestive and absorptive ability of the body has been accelerated. Since the food they take in is digested too quickly, they feel hungry very soon, and eat again. This is exactly the second feature of diabetes: over-eating.

The heat of the spleen also affects the kidneys, giving rise to deficiency and poor astringent ability of the kidneys. This causes patients to urinate a lot. Nutrients are directly discharged out of body through the urine without being fully absorbed. Therefore the body cannot obtain enough nutrition, and patients may become thinner and thinner.

To stay far away from diabetes, one should pay attention to

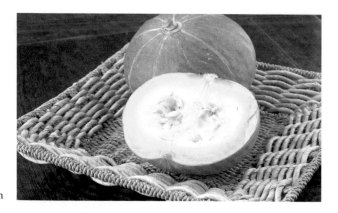

Pumpkin

diet, and especially try to eat a lot of soybean or bean products on a daily basis. This type of food contains a rich amount of protein, inorganic salt and vitamins. Moreover, soybean oil contains a lot of unsaturated fatty acid, which can reduce blood cholesterol and blood triglycerides. The sitosterin contained by soybean oil can also reduce lipids.

Other recommended foods include hull-less oat flour, buckwheat flour, hot oatmeal and corn flour, which contain many micro-elements, Vitamin B and dietary fiber. As shown experimentally, they can slow the rise of blood sugar. Diabetes patients should eat little or no fruit, because fruit contains many carbohydrates, primarily glucose, sucrose and starch. Eating fruit can accelerate digestion and absorption, and can rapidly increase blood sugar. Diabetes patients should eat more vegetables containing dietary fiber, and eat less salt and food with a high content of cholesterol, such as fried food.

In addition to paying attention to diet, diabetes patients should persist in doing moderate physical exercise, for example taking a walk and practicing Taiji (Chinese martial art). This can not only help sufferers to relax both physically and mentally, but also keep them fit. In addition, according to the instruction of doctors, diabetes patients can take drugs to reduce blood sugar, and they should be sure to receive medical examinations at regular intervals.

Keep Slim by Taking Care of the Spleen

Obesity not only affects our health but also impairs our image. In order to keep a slim figure, many people have been fighting fiercely against obesity by continuously trying various slimming drugs, tea and garments. However these usually have little positive effect, and even have caused some negative effects. It is more effective to choose scientific weight-loss methods from a medical perspective, and also to tailor the program to one's physical condition.

According to TCM, obesity is related to the spleen, and the abnormal metabolism of body fluids can give rise to weight problems. As we have learned, the spleen and stomach are seen as the foundation of acquired constitution and the source of the generation and transformation of vital energy and blood. Specifically the spleen is in charge of transportation and transformation. The refined fluids in the body can be transported to internal organs through the spleen. Then they are absorbed or expelled by the body.

When the spleen is in a weak state, its fluid-transporting capacity declines. If fluids cannot be delivered all over the body in time, water dampness and other wastes are deposited in the subcutaneous fat rather than being discharged, thus leading to puffiness. Middle-aged people are more vulnerable to obesity. This is because their spleen function has already been declining gradually, and the transformative and absorptive function of their spleen to fatty and dense food has been weakening slowly. The essence of fluids and grain cannot be delivered properly in the body, and phlegm and fat are accumulated. Moreover middle-aged people who do not often exercise are more likely to become obese.

While more common in middle-aged people, obesity is a problem for some people even since their infancy. Why? This also has something to do with the deficiency of the spleen. Children have relatively weak constitutions. If they continuously

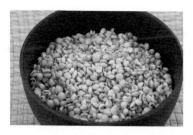

Pearl Barley
With a cold nature and a sweet and light taste, pearl barley can invigorate the spleen and clear heat. It is an age-old recipe for tonifying the spleen and inducing diuresis.

experience infections, the blood in their body would become deficient, and the spleen function would decline, thus giving rise to a constitution marked by spleen deficiency. The spleen is in charge of muscles, so along with the impairment of spleen function, the muscles become flabby, and these children appear obese and swollen. Therefore we can see that the root cause of obesity lies in the spleen.

Then how can we take care of our spleen and prevent obesity from occurring? According to *Yellow Emperor's Inner Canon*, we should protect and nourish our internal organs according to the seasons and time of day. The season of summer and the day's period of Si Time are the best occasions for invigorating the spleen. The saying goes that the spleen "prefers dryness and detests wetness." Therefore it is important to keep the spleen far away from any humid environment, to prevent trouble from pathogenic warmth. We can eat more spleen-invigorating and diuresis-promoting food, such as Chinese dates and beans as well as porridge. Eating porridge in summer can particularly nourish the stomach and invigorate the spleen.

Drooling Shouldn't Be Ignored

Have you ever noticed that you've drooled while sleeping? If you often do so, it is important to pay attention to caring for your spleen.

As *Yellow Emperor's Inner Canon* notes, "Drooling during

sleep indicates a problem with your spleen." How can we interpret this? As discussed previously TCM holds that the spleen is in charge of all muscles. This function of the spleen can be noticed in relation to the mouth, as people suffering from spleen deficiency tend to have flabby facial muscles. Therefore, while asleep, they open their mouths allowing saliva to flow out. In this case drooling is a manifestation of spleen deficiency. The cure for this symptom depends on the specific circumstances of the individual.

Occasional drooling might be caused by improper diet. For example when too much spicy food has been eaten, it may result in the damage of spleen function, heat in the spleen, and too much secretion of saliva. Under such circumstances one needs only to adjust dietary habits, and the symptom will resolve itself soon afterward.

Improper sleeping positions, for example sleeping while bent over a table or sleeping on one's back, tend to bring about drooling. This can be cured with simple changes to position.

Frequent drooling needs to be redressed with a combination of drugs and food therapy. Sufferers can eat porridge with tonic effects, for example a porridge of Chinese dates, or eat starchy foods such as Chinese yam, sweet potato, lotus root and carrot, as well as other spleen-invigorating foods. However patients must use moderation, as over-tonifying can only add burden to the spleen, and can even lead to kidney deficiency.

Drooling can be quite embarrassing and awkward. Traditional

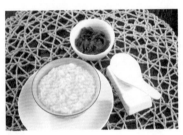

Porridge

Chinese medicine has another tip for changing this bad habit. Since, according to TCM, the tongue is closely related to the spleen, people suffering from spleen deficiency can move their tongue for improvement. To do this exercise, slightly open your lips and stick out your tongue. When it has been stretched to the maximum, maintain this position for five seconds and then withdraw the tongue. Repeat this action 36 times. In another exercise, when tongue is stretched to the maximum, move it from side to side, again for 36 times. After these movements swallow the saliva secreted. This method is quite effective for curing spleen deficiency.

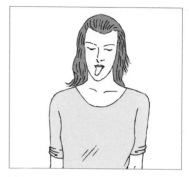

Move tongue to cure spleen deficiency.

Snoring Also Indicates Spleen Disease

Frequently snoring is also a symptom of illness. Medically snoring is termed as "sleep apnea syndrome," and it is a problem for more males than females, by a ratio of six to one. Males also usually begin to snore at an earlier age, usually after the age of 20, while females snore later, mostly after the age of 40.

There are many causes of snoring. Medically it is known that snoring can be caused by hypertension, cardiovascular disease, obesity, diabetes and rheumatoid arthritis. As mentioned previously both diabetes and obesity have something to do with the malfunction of the spleen. Snoring during sleep may also have something to do with the decline of spleen function.

Due to the control of the spleen over the muscles, when there is a problem with the spleen, the muscles become flabby and powerless. In snorers this is manifested by droopy, weak muscles at the uvula, and the jam of pharynx tissues, thus resulting in the collapse of the upper respiratory tract. When the air current passes this narrowed part, an eddy occurs, causing vibration and thus giving rise to a snore. Under serious circumstances the respiratory tract can be fully jammed, thus leading to apnea, and even sudden death, during sleep. So it is important to pay attention to snoring symptoms, and to try the following treatment.

- Pay more attention to protecting and nourishing the spleen in daily life, particularly by eating foods that invigorate or benefit the spleen.
- Do more exercise, especially for the tongue. Exercising the muscle at the tongue reinforces its elasticity. The tongue-stretching and the tongue-wagging methods mentioned above can help to cure snoring.
- Develop healthy habits such as avoiding alcohol, strong tea or coffee before sleep. Maintain a good sleeping position, avoiding lying on the back. Do not take any ethanol-containing drug, sedative or anti-allergic agent, because these make breathing shallow and slow, and make the muscles slacker than usual thus enabling the respiratory tract to be blocked more easily.
- Cure snoring with the help of surgery or instruments, which can effectively and rapidly get rid of the trouble.

You Should Go to the Doctor When ...
If any of the following seven circumstances occurs when one has been snoring, a doctor should be consulted:

1. Still feeling very tired in spite of an overnight sleep.
2. Repeatedly waking up due to a feeling of suffocation at night; tossing about involuntarily; or even fainting or twitching.
3. Suffering from headache, parched mouth and dry tongue after waking up.
4. Always feeling sleepy or dozing off in the daytime; especially if one is falling asleep at work or while driving vehicles.
5. Remaining irritable and bad-tempered; having a higher blood pressure after waking up.
6. Suffering from distraction or memory issues.
7. Suffering from penile erectile dysfunction or decline of sexual desire.

Prevent Excessive Thinking from Impairing Spleen

According to *Yellow Emperor's Inner Canon*, people have five emotions: joy, anger, sadness, thinking and fear. These five emotions correspond with TCM's five organs: heart, liver, lung, kidney and spleen. The spleen is the organ that corresponds with thinking. Although thinking is a normal activity, excessive thinking, or over-analyzing or worry, can lead to the stagnation of energy and the imbalance of transportation and transformation, thus giving rise to disease.

Why are unnecessary anxiety and sentimentality harmful to the spleen? If we always worry about this or that, having changeable emotions and too many thoughts whenever anything occurs, this may result in the loss of appetite and exert a negative influence on the spleen and kidney. Along with the stagnation of spleen energy and indigestion, this can lead to weight loss. Excessive thinking adds burden to the brain, and impairs spleen health in the long run.

Shouldn't we think about anything? The answer, absolutely, is "yes." Normal "thinking" is necessary; otherwise we cannot solve problems with our work or life. Medically, not "thinking" would make us dull, lazy and obese. But thinking should be kept within a limit.

How should people who think too much invigorate their spleen? Poria cocos, which can be used as a drug and therapeutic food, is recommended. As a parasitic fungus plant on the root of pine, poria cocos is shaped like a sweet potato, has a black brown husk, a white or pink interior, a sweet and light taste, and a mild nature. It has a mild medicinal property, and is effective in invigorating the spleen. The ancient TCM text, *Herbal Classic*, notes that poria cocos "can nurture our soul if taken for a long time."

Powdered poria cocos can be found at some drugstores or in specialty herbal shops. Poria cocos can clear dampness, promote diuresis, benefit the spleen and stomach, and pacify the mind and soothe the nerves. You can take it after mixing it with boiled water or milk, or make a porridge with it; the latter two can produce a better effect.

How to Exercise the Spleen Meridian

People in ancient times paid great attention to climatic condition, favorable location and community. Only by conforming to the laws of nature could they gain the greatest harvest. If we now follow these natural laws, we must exercise the Spleen Meridian at Si Time (9 to 11 a.m.), instead of earlier or later. This is because our vital energy and blood are flowing past the Spleen Meridian at Si Time, and this meridian is in its prime. Earlier than that, the spleen has not yet begun to work; later, the spleen works much less efficiently and no obvious effect of exercising can be achieved.

Nowadays many health experts, especially in yoga, advocate a method of "grasping the ground with the toes," a recommendation which correlates to TCM. This is because the

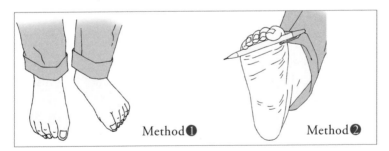

Method❶   Method❷

Ground-Grasping Method

❶ Slightly hunching the dorsum of feet, and bending inward the ten toes of our feet, as if grasping the ground, which can exercise our spleen meridian.

❷ Lying on the back, and trying to grab some small articles with toes, which can exercise the meridians and collaterals of our feet.

Spleen Meridian passes the hallux (big) toe, and the Stomach Meridian passes the second and third toes. By exercising our toes we can invigorate the spleen and nourish the stomach.

The following recommended exercise is simple. While standing exert pressure on the shin, and push the toes evenly downward, as if trying to grasp the ground. Hold for five seconds, then take a rest and begin this process all over again. Repeat 50 times at the beginning, then gradually increase to 100 repetitions.

You can also do an exercise lying down by putting some small articles on the bed (key, pen or small ball, for example), and trying to grasp them with the toes. This is not only interesting but also capable of fully exercising the meridians and collaterals on the feet.

In addition to the above-mentioned methods, tapping the Spleen Meridian is recommended. Press painful spots (if any) for a longer time, which also exercises the Spleen Meridian. In fact there are many methods; it is important to choose the method that best suits you and practice it daily.

For busy people who do not have much time for exercise, the following seated exercise is recommended: the "4" leg technique. Press the thigh with the ankle of the other foot. Maintaining this comfortable position will relax you both physically and mentally. More importantly you can massage the Spleen Meridian through such a seated posture. The Spleen Meridian goes upward exactly from the Yinbai point at the hallux toe, along the mid-line of the inner shin, and to the inner thigh, before going into our

Exercising the Spleen Meridian with the "4" Leg Technique

This seated posture provides an ideal position for massaging the Spleen Meridian. Pressing the thigh with the ankle of the other foot, tap upward along the route of the meridian.

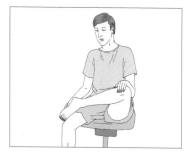

abdominal cavity. So this posture is convenient for massaging the meridian. Pat upward along the route with an appropriate force. You can slightly exert the strength of your leg at the same time. Tap each side for about ten minutes (or longer if you have time).

Remember that it is best to tap the meridian from 9 to 11 a.m., and that exercise can be done at any place. By maintaining a regular practice of exercising and choosing the most suitable method, it is easy to keep healthy.

Protect and Nourish Spleen According to Season

Previously we learned that *Yellow Emperor's Inner Canon* states that health promotion should conform to the change of seasons, and the liver, heart, spleen, lung and kidney correspond with spring, summer, late summer, autumn and winter respectively. Therefore it is the most timely to protect and nourish the spleen during the sixth month of the Chinese lunar calendar.

Late summer refers to the period when the summer has come to its end but the autumn has not yet arrived. In this period yang energy begins to change from release to collection, and all living things on earth grow lushly. Yin and yang energy on the earth are exchanged with each other and there is liveliness everywhere.

It is an ancient belief that all living things should preserve yang energy in summer to meet the requirement of growth. For example plants should accumulate a lot of energy at this time so as to bear rich fruits in autumn. In addition, in this period of the year, the spleen has the strongest energy and vigor, and the body absorbs the largest amount of vital essence from Mother Nature. The vital essence is stored in the spleen. Enough yang energy must be stored in the spleen so as to lay a foundation for the arrival of autumn and winter.

In summer we can go to bed later and get up earlier. However it is important to take care not to become upset and irritable, and to maintain an optimistic mood. In this way yang energy in the body can move smoothly, keeping us quite energetic. In addition, we should also pay attention to diet, trying to eat light, mild and easily digestible food. It is recommended to eat foods that can invigorate the spleen and promote diuresis, such as pearl barley, vigna umbellata and buckwheat. Do not eat a lot of raw, cold and oily food, and overall one should not eat and drink too much. Take care to prevent dampness, and avoid living in a shady and cold environment. Keep windows open in most cases to maintain indoor air ventilation.

Folk Prescriptions

1. Mix 10 g raw mashed garlic and a little sugar and vinegar. Taken before a regular meal, this can not only refresh the spleen and invigorate the stomach, but also prevent intestinal disease.

2. Mix 20 g hawthorn chips, 5 g sliced ginger. Take to promote digestion and whet appetite.

3. Mix 125 g caraway, 50 g jellyfish, and some salt, sugar and vinegar. This aromatic mixture can whet the appetite and invigorate the spleen.

4. Medicinal porridges to protect the spleen and invigorate the stomach:

- 50 g lotus seed, 50 g dolichos seeds, 50 g pearl barley
- 20 g white fungus, 10 g lily bulb, 20 g mung beans, 100 g glutinous rice
- 50 g Chinese yam, 50 g poria cocos, 250 g stir-fried polished round-grained rice

Prevent Minor Illness by Regulating Spleen Meridian

We can prevent and cure a variety of diseases by regulating the Spleen Meridian. There are a total of 21 acupoints on the Spleen Meridian, including the Taibai, Sanyinjiao, Yinbai and Xuehai

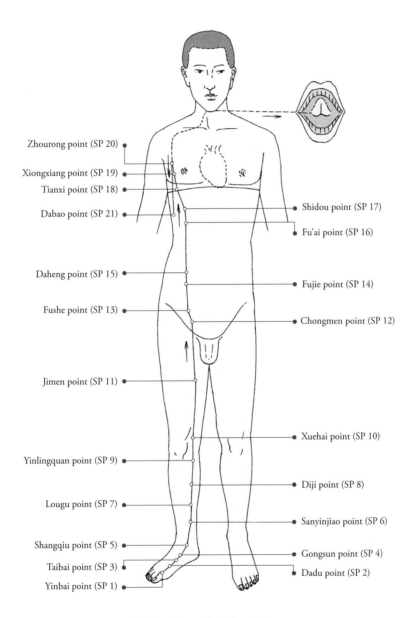

Zhourong point (SP 20)

Xiongxiang point (SP 19)

Tianxi point (SP 18)

Dabao point (SP 21)

Shidou point (SP 17)

Fu'ai point (SP 16)

Daheng point (SP 15)

Fujie point (SP 14)

Fushe point (SP 13)

Chongmen point (SP 12)

Jimen point (SP 11)

Xuehai point (SP 10)

Yinlingquan point (SP 9)

Diji point (SP 8)

Lougu point (SP 7)

Sanyinjiao point (SP 6)

Shangqiu point (SP 5)

Gongsun point (SP 4)

Taibai point (SP 3)

Dadu point (SP 2)

Yinbai point (SP 1)

Taiyin Spleen Meridian of Foot

points, which are very important in controlling the spleen and preserving health.

The Taiyin Spleen Meridian of Foot starts at the Yinbai point at the tip of the hallux toe, continuing along the inside of this toe and connecting the instep and sole. It goes upward to the rear of the ankle, and then passes the inner calf, and along the rear edge of the shin bone. It proceeds upward to the front edge of the inner thigh, enters the abdomen, becomes part of the spleen, connects with the stomach, and goes further upward, passing the thoracic diaphragm (diaphragm muscle). It enters the throat, links with the root of the tongue and scatters below the tongue.

Taibai Point

The Taibai point is located on the inner edge of the foot, at the depression between the inside and outside of the rear lower part of the hallux toe. This point can cure stomachache, abdominal distension, vomiting, hiccup, borborygmus, diarrhea, dysentery, constipation, beriberi and anal fistula. Often massaging or practicing moxibustion on this point can help in invigorating the spleen and getting rid of diseases.

Sanyinjiao Point

This acupoint is located in the inner shin, 3 cun above the top of the inner ankle and behind the inner edge of the shin bone. This point can cure irregular menstruation, dysmenorrheal, leucorrhoea with reddish discharge, impotence, premature ejaculation, phallodynia, urodialysis, edema, muscular soreness, abdominal distension, eczema and urticaria. Massage

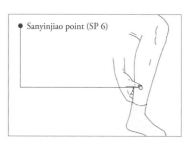

Sanyinjiao point (SP 6)

Pressing and Kneading Sanyinjiao Point

This acupoint is located in the inner shin, 3 cun above the top of the inner ankle, and behind the inner edge of the shin bone.

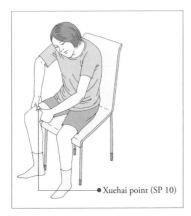

Pressing and Kneading Xuehai Point

This acupoint is located on the inner thigh, 2 cun above the inner end of the bottom of the patella, and at the inner end of the quadriceps femoris.

or practice moxibustion on this acupoint to prevent and cure diseases. However women should take care not to stimulate this acupoint during menstruation; otherwise too much menstruation could possibly occur.

Yinbai Point

This acupoint is located about 0.1 cun away from the inner toenail corner of the hallux toe. Using the method of moxibustion or applying ground medicines as a paste is most effective for this acupoint. It can cure hypermenorrhea, metrorrhagia and metrostaxis, hematochezia, hematuria, abdominal distension, insanity, nightmares and infantile convulsion.

Xuehai Point

To find the location of this acupoint, sit on a chair with bent knees. You will find this acupoint located in the inner thigh, 2 cun over the inner end of the bottom of the patella, and at the hunch of the inner end of the quadriceps femoris. The Xuehai point is in charge of irregular menstruation, metrorrhagia and metrostaxis, amenorrhea, urticaria, eczema and erysipelas. Press this acupoint with the thumb with due force for 3 to 5 minutes, massaging each of the thighs in turn or at the same time, once a day.

Chapter Seven

Wu Time (11 a.m. to 1 p.m.)
Heart Meridian in Its Prime

At Wu Time (11 a.m. to 1 p.m.) the Shaoyin Heart Meridian of Hand (Heart Meridian) begins to work. *Yellow Emperor's Inner Canon* advises, "Go to bed when your yang energy is exhausted; wake up when your yin energy is exhausted." This means that getting some sleep at Wu Time is the best regimen. Sleep at this time can nurture your soul and build your body.

After working the whole morning, we have consumed a huge amount of energy and stamina. If we can take a nap for a while, we will reserve enough energy and vigor to continue our studies or labor for the whole afternoon. However many people are unable or neglect to nap at noon because of being busy. This leads to feeling dizzy, sleepy and fuzzy-headed in the afternoon, and affects the efficiency of work and study.

From the perspective of yin-yang harmonization, from the time we wake in the early morning until 11 a.m., the yang energy in the body rises continuously to its peak. After this time, yang energy begins to weaken, and yin energy begins to grow. Having a good rest at this time replenishes the energy in our body to the maximum.

Therefore it is best to take a nap at noon, following the laws of nature, so as to ensure that we have plentiful energy afterward. Even if one cannot go to sleep at this time, it is helpful just to close the eyes for a short repose.

According to TCM, at Wu Time, the internal heat of the body reaches its peak. Sleep at this time is the most effective way to reduce this internal heat. When one is at rest, the mind becomes more peaceful, the pulse smoother and steadier, and internal heat declines slowly. When we have excessive internal heat, it may erupt like a volcano in the long run, thus giving rise to oral ulcer, irritability, insomnia and dreaminess.

A noontime nap can also nourish the blood. The heart is in charge of the blood vessels, and it is also in charge of sweating, which stems from the blood. If we move about at noon in hot summer, we will feel very hot and perspire profusely, and too much perspiration impairs yin and blood. A short nap can restrain sweat and nourish the blood, thus bringing many benefits to the body.

For better health it is best to follow the rhythms of nature, and to take a nap at midday.

Replenish Energy and Blood by Taking a Nap

We have seen that taking a nap at noon is vital, but what should we pay attention to at this nap-time? How long should the noon nap last? In what position should we take this nap?

There is advice in an age-old saying: "A sound sleep at Zi Time; a short nap at Wu Time." There is a clear distinction between these two kinds of sleep. At Zi Time (midnight), we have already fallen into a state of deep sleep. At Wu Time (in the daytime), we need only to take a short nap.

According to expert analysis, people go to sleep most easily eight hours after getting up in the early morning or eight hours before going to bed at night. Based on due calculation, this is about 1 p.m. Traditional wisdom holds that alertness is in a period of natural decline at this time. Taking a short nap around this time is an ideal way to relax the body. However the duration of this

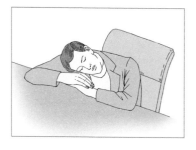

Wrong Nap Position
Taking a nap by bending over a desk restricts our meridians, collaterals and nerves, as well as blood and oxygen circulation, leading to a number of adverse symptoms upon waking.

nap should be controlled, lasting between ten minutes and one hour. We can also make due adjustment to the duration according to actual conditions. For example very strong and vigorous people can take a nap of ten minutes to half an hour, while children and elderly people can take a nap of about an hour. Even if one's schedule is tight, one should rest for at least ten minutes, or close the eyes in order to nurture the soul.

You must also choose a suitable position, otherwise you will not only fail to relax the body, but may actually create discomfort. Many office workers choose to take a nap by bending over their desks. In fact this is harmful for the body, because this position oppresses the meridians, collaterals and nerves. It also hinders blood circulation, results in blood and oxygen deficiency in the brain, and brings about dizziness, blurred vision, weakness and other symptoms upon waking up. Therefore, rather than bending over a desk, it is best to take a noontime nap by leaning back in a chair. When at home, lying on a sofa or bed is an ideal choice.

Light, mild and non-oily food is recommended for lunch, and it is important not to eat too much food at noon. Oily food can increase the viscosity of blood, and worsen any lesion of the coronary artery. Eating too much food can add digestive burden to the stomach. Drinking a glass of water after waking up will replenish blood volume and properly dilute blood viscosity. Then it is good to take up some light activities, for example going for a walk.

It is also inadvisable to take a nap by lying on one side with a hand supporting the head, or with both hands crossed behind

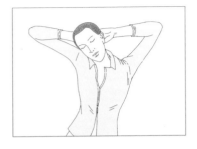

Wrong Nap Position
Using one's hands as a pillow when napping will not only fail to lead to relaxation but may also cause health complications.

the head. Using the hands as a pillow can easily pull the muscles and displace the thoracic diaphragm, thus leading to the rise of abdominal pressure; in the long run, it may possibly result in the congestion, edema and irritation of mucous membranes in the esophagus and reflux esophagitis. In addition, this sleeping posture can affect breathing, thus leading to such symptoms as chest oppression and fatigue.

Several Tips for Lunch

Lunch can be the most important meal, providing 40% of the total energy consumed over the whole day. Therefore we should pay attention to making the right choices at lunch.

The most important consideration is the timing for lunch. Most people who nap at midday have a habit of taking this nap immediately after having lunch, which is in fact harmful for the body. It is better to reverse the order, and take a nap before lunch. Taking a nap after having lunch affects digestion, prevents the absorption of food, and may even result in indigestion or gastric diseases. In addition, the blood gathers in the stomach after lunch, thus leading to a short supply of blood to the brain. Therefore if we nap after lunch, we may feel dizzy and uncomfortable after waking up.

It is best to arrange lunch time between 12:30 p.m. and 1 p.m., when the Heart Meridian is on duty. At 1 p.m. the small intestine begins to work. After lunch the food passes the spleen and stomach, and will arrive at the small intestine at exactly the right time. The small intestine continues to absorb, digest and decompose the food, and they can work much more efficiently at this time, when the energy and blood flow past the Small Intestine Meridian. As a result the absorbed food will be fully digested, the essence of the food delivered to the internal organs, and the waste filtered and expelled from the body. Therefore having lunch at this time will help in avoiding many intestinal and gastric diseases, as well as ensure normal metabolism and considerably reduce the chance of obesity.

For a healthy lunch, choose food with a high content of fiber and a low content of oil, salt and sugar. Staple food of 150 to 200 grams should be eaten to meet the requirements for inorganic salt and vitamins. A sizeable portion of vegetables (200–250 grams) and a moderate amount of meat, egg and fish (50–100 grams) should be eaten. Avoid food with low nutritional value, such as instant noodles.

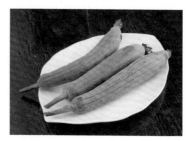

Luffa

Use Quietness to Nourish the Heart

The heart is in charge of our spirit and will, according to the record of *Yellow Emperor's Inner Canon*, and it is the sovereign governing all internal organs and coordinating the whole body. Therefore it is of vital importance to protect and nourish the heart. *Yellow Emperor's Inner Canon* goes on to state that we should maintain a sedate spirit and a placid state of mind every day, thus leaving no opportunity for invasion by disease. It emphasizes the great wisdom of nourishing the heart with quietness.

Traditional Chinese medicine lays a particular stress on

resting to restore mental tranquility. Maintain a peaceful state of mind while nourishing the heart can relieve and prevent diseases. For example when a person is ill (especially when a person has just recovered from dangerous illness), the doctor will require this patient to relax for recuperation. This is because a great deal of yang energy in the body will have been lost, weakening it after illness. When one has good relaxation for recuperation, the yang energy in the body gradually increases, the yin and the yang are reconciled gradually, and the resistant capacity of the body to diseases increases slowly, which is conducive to the quick recovery of health.

Methods for Relaxation-Based Recuperation

1. Sleeping: When asleep people can relax their body and mind thoroughly.

2. Sitting quietly: Often sitting with crossed legs can nuture the mind and soul.

3. Relaxation-based recuperation exercise: This type of exercise has such efficacies as getting rid of illness, building health and prolonging life. Sit or lie down, with feet shoulder-width and both hands laid flat. First breathe air deeply into the pubic region, rolling up the tongue until it presses the palate while

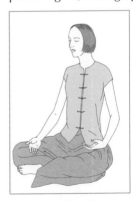

**Relaxation-Based
Recuperation Exercise**

inhaling. Silently say "I" in the mind at the same time. Next silently say "release" at the same time as releasing the tongue. Finally, silently say "silent" in mind, and guard the lower torso area with your mind, thinking protective thoughts. Repeat this for 15 to 30 minutes. You will feel a gust of plentiful air slowly spreading from the pubic region, the blood in the four limbs flowing very fast, and your palms glowing because of the smooth circulation of energy and blood.

During the whole process you should concentrate your attention, and then you will feel relaxed all over upon completion. Practice the exercise twice a day.

Cure Depression by Regulating Heart Meridian

Our guide, *Yellow Emperor's Inner Canon*, tells us that the heart is in charge of our internal spirit. Any problem with the spirit has something to do with the Heart Meridian. If energy in the heart is smooth, we will feel energetic, vigorous and high-spirited; otherwise we will feel depressed and negative.

Depression is a common mental disorder, and sufferers become low-spirited, passive, pessimistic, slow-minded, self-critical, forgetful and sleepless. They may become hypochondriacs, may experience discomfort all over the body, and even feel suicidal. The occurrence of depression is often related to mental stress. For example office workers may often force themselves to fulfill tasks within the shortest time, and if there is any delay, or if they fail to fulfill the tasks in time, they become extremely anxious and chastise themselves. In the long run this leads to withdrawal and reticence, low-spirits and depression.

Depression is mostly related to moods, which can be regulated with the help of the Heart Meridian. The Shenmen point is an important acupoint on the Shaoyin Heart Meridian of Hand. It is also a "source acupoint" where many meridians and collaterals, vital energy and blood converge. This acupoint acts as an important "switch" for regulating the energy of the heart. Turning on this "switch" can not only clear the Heart Meridian, but also regulate the energy and blood in our heart. A smooth Heart Meridian along with sufficient energy and blood brings a good mood, and eliminates depression and negativity.

The Shenmen point is located at the depression below the cross striation on the inner wrist. To find the point, bend your

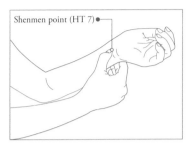

Shenmen point (HT 7)

Massage Shenmen point.

arms letting your palms face upward. There is a small circular bone at the lateral end of the hypothenar with a tendon behind this bone. The intersection between the tendon and the cross striation of the wrists is the Shenmen point.

To use this acupoint, stretch one hand out straight, and press the Shenmen point with the index finger of the other hand for point-and-pressure. Press and release for about five minutes. Then change to the other hand. Practice this once or twice a day. Perform this preferably at noon when the Heart Meridian is in its prime. This method helps to regulate the heart and soul, get rid of depression, and promote sleep.

Judge Heart Disease by Complexion

According to traditional Chinese medicine, any damage within the body will inevitably be reflected on the body surface. Therefore we can get to know heart diseases by looking at the face and the five facial organs. If traces of heart disease can be observed on the face, we can make an early discovery of these diseases, and take prompt steps toward a cure.

1. Observing facial complexion: You can ask a doctor perform this observation, or you can carefully observe your complexion with a mirror at home. If your facial skin looks ruddy and glossy, this indicates good heart function and you need not worry. However if your face, especially the cheek, is dark red, you should take care, because this is a sign of rheumatic heart disease. If your face is dark brown or dark purple, do not treat this lightly, because this may indicate chronic cardiac failure and late pulmonary heart disease. In addition, pay more attention to

red blood streaks. People with suboptimal heart function often have faces covered with streaks, which indicate that something is wrong with their blood cycle system.

2. Observing the five facial organs: Some reactions of these organs also correlate with heart diseases. Based on careful observation, we can prevent and cure heart diseases in advance.

- Ears: TCM believes that the "heart has an outlet in the ears." By observing symptoms on the ears, we can notice some clues as to heart function. Clinical observation has found that a continuous crease can often be discovered on the skin in the front of the ears of many patients with heart diseases. If you have this symptom, you must pay close attention, because this probably indicates that the coronary artery is hardening or has already hardened. At this time congestion would occur to the blood vessels in the body. When the congestion of the atherosclerosis of the coronary artery reaches 60%, angina or myocardial infarction may occur, as well as various cardiovascular and cerebrovascular diseases. In addition, earache and tinnitus are also signs of early stages of heart disease. So if you suddenly feel a pain or buzz in your ears, consult a doctor as soon as possible.

- Nose: According to TCM, the base of the nose bridge between the eyes can indicate heart condition. Therefore some heart problems can also be discovered in advance by observing the nose. If a cross striation occurs at the nose, one should take care, because this indicates that the heart rate is irregular or that something else is wrong with the heart. In addition, a red nose tip is also a bad sign. Unless due to weather factors, if the nose tip has swollen or reddened, this may indicate that heart disease has become aggravated.

- Tongue: The tongue of a healthy person is pink. The whitening of the tongue indicates insufficient blood supply to the cardiac muscle. The frequent darkening and empurpling of the tongue tip indicate undesirable blood circulation and viscous blood, which may tend to trigger blood congestion as well as cardiovascular and cerebrovascular diseases. The appearance of many small red spots on the tip of tongue may be a sign of myocarditis. We should also pay attention when deep vertical striations occur on the tip of the tongue, because this forebodes the advent of heart disease.

The above-mentioned, which are some common facial manifestations of heart disease, are provided here for reference only. Please note that one cannot judge heart disease by only one or two of these symptoms. It is important to observe these symptoms comprehensively, and ask experienced doctors to make a definite diagnosis.

Relationship of Meridians and Collaterals to Heart Problems

Yellow Emperor's Inner Canon states that the heart is linked with meridians and collaterals in a system of mutual reliance and influence. In other words if any problem occurs to the meridians and collaterals, it will exert due influence on the heart.

1. Heart Meridian: Starting from the heart, one branch of the Heart Meridian runs through the diaphragm, then goes downward and links with the small intestine. The other branch goes out obliquely from the armpit, passes through the inner arms, links with the center of the palm, and arrives at the tip of the middle finger. If there is any problem along this meridian (i.e. pain or numb distention in the inner arms, dryness in the throat, suppression in the chest or ache in the heart), then there may be a problem with the heart.

2. Lung Meridian: *Yellow Emperor's Inner Canon* describes many symptoms of diseases attributed to the lung. As one of these symptoms, chest suppression is in fact a problem with the heart that manifests along the Lung Meridian. Any problem with the Lung

Meridian results in disturbed operation of energy and blood as well as the undesirable circulation of blood, thus triggering heart diseases.

3. Spleen Meridian: Since the Spleen Meridian passes through the heart, any problem with this meridian can be manifested directly at the heart. The spleen is in charge of transportation and transformation. If there is discomfort along the meridian, it cannot transport enough "essence of water and grains" (i.e. nutritional substances) to other internal organs including the heart. If your heart cannot obtain sufficient nutrition, you may feel flustered, your heartbeat would be accelerated, your mood would become fidgety, and your heart would ache faintly. In addition, the spleen has the function of ensuring that blood runs in vessels and prevents it from overflowing. If the Spleen Meridian is blocked, energy is unable to control blood, and blood flow is no longer smooth, thus affecting circulation and impairing heart function.

4. Stomach Meridian: The Stomach Meridian also runs through the heart. Problems with this meridian affect the digestion and absorption of food. This may lead to malnutrition, hunger, feeling flustered and accelerated heartbeat. On the contrary, eating too much is also harmful for the heart. If there is too much food in the stomach, most blood in the body is transferred to the stomach. This means that insufficient blood would be supplied to the heart, causing it to palpitate irregularly. In addition stomach-cold and stomach-heat would also be conducted to the heart, thus triggering heart-heat.

5. Kidney Meridian: The kidney is where energy and essence are stored, and the so-called "spirit" stems from the kidney. If the kidneys suffer from a serious loss of energy and essence, the heart will also be affected. Deficiency or exhaustion of kidney essence leads to arrhythmia, often accompanied with heart palpitation or a noticeable pause of heartbeat. If this recurs it can reduce the blood discharge of heart, decrease power, cause head dizziness and chest suppression, and aggravate any existing angina or cardiac failure.

6. Pericardium Meridian: The pericardium is a thin film

wrapped around the outside of the heart. The Pericardium Meridian is an important one, connecting the pericardium and heart. Heart diseases at their earliest stages are manifested through this meridian. Patients often feel chest suppression, anxiety and nausea. Often massaging and exercising the Pericardium Meridian can prevent heart diseases.

It is important to pay more attention to observation of your body's condition every day. If you experience any pain or discomfort in the meridians and collaterals, you must not treat this lightly. It is probable that the injury to the meridian or collateral is related to a heart problem. Therefore it is best to receive a medical examination as soon as possible.

How to Exercise the Heart Meridian

According to *A Book on Longevity*, an important Taoist text dating to the Southern and Northern Dynasties in China (420–589), "We can achieve longevity by attaining mental tranquility through full relaxation and exercising our body through movements." This advice still holds; in order to nourish the heart, we should not only fully relax ourselves but also do proper exercises. We can nourish the heart and get rid of disease by pressing and kneading key acupoints on the Shaoyin Heart Meridian of Hand.

This meridian starts from the heart and separates into two branches. One branch internally runs through the trunk and then goes downward, running through the diaphragm and linking with the small intestine. The other branch (also a main branch) externally runs through the trunk, passing through the lungs from the heart. It goes out obliquely from the armpit, and then runs along the inner arms and the center of the elbow. This branch enters the palm from the end of the protuberant bone behind the palm, and arrives at the end along the radialis of the little finger.

The Jiquan point, Shaohai point and Shenmen point are

major acupoints on the Shaoyin Heart Meridian of Hand. In daily practice, frequently pressing and kneading these acupoints can soothe the nerves and nourish the heart.

Jiquan Point

The Jiquan point is located under the armpit. If you bend at the elbow and press the back of the head with the palms, you will find a place of artery pulsation at the center of the armpit. Press and knead this acupoint with the end of the thumb for three to five minutes using due force. Then shift to the other side. Often pressing and kneading this acupoint can soothe and activate the meridians; regulate heart energy; relieve symptoms such as heartache, chest suppression and dry mouth; and prevent coronary heart disease and pulmonary disease.

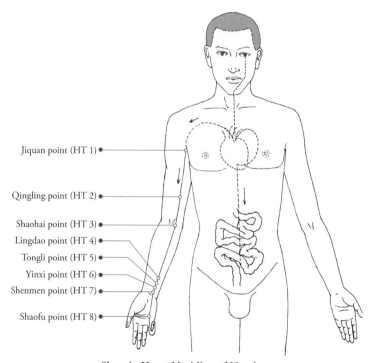

Jiquan point (HT 1)
Qingling point (HT 2)
Shaohai point (HT 3)
Lingdao point (HT 4)
Tongli point (HT 5)
Yinxi point (HT 6)
Shenmen point (HT 7)
Shaofu point (HT 8)

Shaoyin Heart Meridian of Hand

Shaohai Point

Also named the "Qujie point," the Shaohai point is found in the inner arm. If the elbow is bent, the midpoint between the inner cross striation of the elbow and the inner epicondyle of humerus is the exact location of this acupoint. Press and knead this point with due force with one hand, and shift to the other side after three minutes. Massaging this acupoint has an excellent curative effect for symptoms including heartache, numb and shaky arms, axillary and side-rib pain, forgetfulness and insomnia.

Shenmen Point

The Shenmen point is located on the outer edge of the cross striation of the wrist, at the radial depression of the ulnar wrist flexor tendon. Pinch and press this point with the tip of the thumb for three to five minutes, and then shift to the other hand. With frequent practice this exercise can cure problems such as angina, acrotism, neurosis, hysteria, schizophrenia, epigastric pain and indigestion.

Massaging the Heart Meridian

In addition to pressing and kneading acupoints, massaging the Heart Meridian can also be beneficial. Push the Heart Meridian at the base of the middle finger (where it connects to the palm). Perform a clockwise rotation from the fingertip to the base. This method can nourish the heart and soothe the mind.

Pushing it in a linear way (from tip to base) can quench heart fire. This method can also cure oral ulcers, heart fire and heat, and deficiency of heart blood.

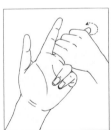

Nourishing the Heart Meridian

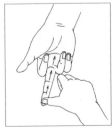

Quenching Heart-Heat

Chapter Eight

Wei Time (1 p.m. to 3 p.m.)
Small Intestine Meridian in Its Prime

At Wei Time (1 p.m. to 3 p.m.) the Taiyang Small Intestine Meridian of Hand (Small Intestine Meridian) begins to work, giving the body a strong ability to digest and absorb food. *Yellow Emperor's Inner Canon* describes the small intestine as an organ of accepting, digesting and absorbing nutritional substances. Its major function is to distinguish the essential part of food and transform it into energy, before distributing it to other organs of the body.

Although the small intestine, spleen and stomach are all digestive organs, they have their respective duties. Just like the production line in a food processing factory, raw material can become food only after several procedures. First, food arrives at the mouth, where it is ground with the help of teeth and saliva before entering the spleen and stomach. The food is further processed in the spleen and stomach.

The stomach is just like a grinding and a mixing machine. After it completes this task, the job of "transformation" is assigned to the small intestine. It carries out "fine processing." The difference between the small intestine and spleen/stomach is as follows: the small intestine absorbs nutritional substances more meticulously, "classifies" the food, absorbs its essence, transforms it into energy, and transports it to the internal organs to maintain the body's normal activities. The remains of the food are delivered to the large intestine, which continues to absorb moisture before transporting waste to the anus to be discharged from the body. This is the path of food through body, a process in which the small intestine plays a vital role.

Wei Time is the time when the Small Intestine Meridian works. During this time, when energy and blood pass this meridian, the small intestine has the strongest ability to digest food, absorb nutrition and pass along waste. When one eats an appropriate lunch, the small intestine obtains enough nutritional supply, and the energy and blood within the small intestine are sufficient.

The Small Intestine Meridian links with the heart and has a close relationship with the Heart Meridian. If the Small Intestine Meridian has sufficient energy and blood, the heart will have a strong ability to supply blood. When the Small Intestine Meridian has smooth energy and blood, we feel extremely energetic. Otherwise the energy and blood supply of the whole body is affected, and extra burden added to the heart and its meridian. Over the long term, eating improperly at lunch leads to insufficient energy and blood of the small intestine. If one cannot absorb enough nutrition, physical constitution declines, leaving the body open to the attack of various diseases.

Small Intestine Meridian Defects May Impair Ears

Deafness is a kind of hearing disorder with degrees of severity; some patients cannot hear sounds outside perfectly, while those with serious or full deafness cannot hear sounds outside at all. Another hearing disorder is tinnitus, in which unusual sounds (usually ringing) occur in the ears without any external stimulation. Tinnitus is often an omen of deafness. Patients with serious tinnitus and deafness often experience difficulty in working, living and sleeping normally, and they may face problems with interpersonal relationships as well as some mental

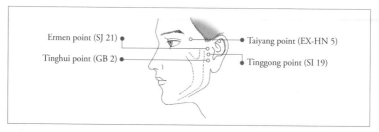

Ermen point (SJ 21)

Tinghui point (GB 2)

Taiyang point (EX-HN 5)

Tinggong point (SI 19)

Tinggong Point

disorders such as neurasthenia and insomnia.

There are many causes of deafness and tinnitus, including environmental noise pollution, drug effects, work pressure, fatigue, insufficient sleep and heredity. In addition, there is an important cause that tends to be ignored: impairments of our meridians and collaterals.

There are many ear-related meridians and collaterals, of which the Small Intestine Meridian is one. The health of the ears is closely related to this meridian. It extends from the Shaoze point on the outer fingers to the Tinggong point on the ears.

The Tinggong point is a vital acupoint on the Small Intestine Meridian. Many ear diseases are related to this point. It is located on the part of ears close to the face, at the depression in front of the antilobium when the mouth is opened, in the depression of the parallel gap of the tragus and slightly below the Ermen point. Pointing and kneading this acupoint can help with ear problems such as deafness, tinnitus and hearing loss.

Exercises for Ear Health

1. You may sit upright, lie on your back or recline. Accurately locating the acupoint, place the tips of both index fingers on the Tinggong points on the right and left ear. Knead and press with due force for one to two minutes. This can help in improving hearing and eyesight and refreshing yourself.

2. Massage the base of the ears by first rubbing your hands together to produce heat, and then clamping each ear with the

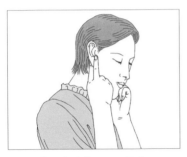

Massaging the Tinggong Point
Placing index fingers of both hands on Tinggong point of both ears. Kneading and pressing the point for 1 to 2 minutes.

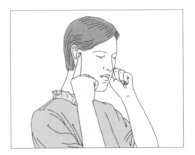

Massaging the Base of the Ears
After chafing both hands, clamping the root of both ears with the index finger and middle finger of both hands. Massaging the root of ears up and down with due force for 3 to 5 minutes.

index and middle finger. Massage up and down with due force for three to five minutes. This method stimulates such acupoints as Ermen, Tinggong and Tinghui, thus preventing and curing earache, tinnitus and otitis.

3. After rubbing hands together, stroke both auricles on all sides for three minutes. This method can prevent and cure all ear diseases.

In addition to massaging major acupoints on the Small Intestine Meridian, increased daily physical exercise, especially of the hands, neck and head, is recommended. Since the Small Intestine Meridian passes directly through these parts, fully exercising them can soothe and activate the meridians and collaterals, clear the Small Intestine Meridian, and prevent such diseases as deafness and tinnitus.

Cure Certain Heart Problems through Small Intestine Meridian

Such symptoms as face flush, rapid heartbeat, chest oppression and shortness of breath often happen to certain people from 2 to 3 p.m. These are external manifestations of heart problems according to *Yellow Emperor's Inner Canon*. The Small Intestine Meridian is closely related to the heart, starting from the heart and integrating with the Heart Meridian.

Early signs of problems with the heart can be noticed in the Small Intestine Meridian. Because the Small Intestine Meridian is at its peak around 2 to 3 p.m., we can cure the above symptoms most effectively by regulating the meridian during this time.

The heart corresponds with heat (or fire) in TCM's "Five Elements" systems. The heart is in charge of blood vessels. If heart-heat is too strong, blood heat goes upward, making the face unusually red or purple. Heart-heat may become too vigorous if we are overly emotional (whether it be excitement, happiness, sadness or other feelings), if we eat certain foods (for example fried, barbecued or spicy food), or if we do not sleep optimally or often suffer from insomnia.

Under such circumstances, we can clear our meridians and collaterals by regulating the Small Intestine Meridian, leading heart-heat into the small intestine where it can be discharged from the body.

How should we regulate the Small Intestine Meridian? There are two important acupoints on this meridian, namely the Houxi and Qiangu points.

- Houxi point: To find this point, make a loose fist. You will find the Houxi point at the ulnar palm cross-striation behind the metacarpal joint of the ring finger, and at the boundary that connects the palm and the back of the hand.

- Qiangu point: It is located below the Houxi point, namely at the depression on the outer edge of the first joint that connects the palm with the ring finger.

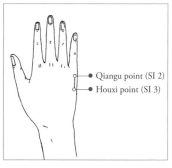

Houxi Point and Qiangu Point

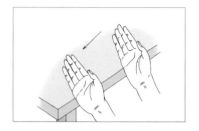

"Cutting Vegetables" Exercise
With the hand held vertically as a "knife," make a cutting action on the edge of table with the pinky side of the hand.

To stimulate these two acupoints, you can try the exercise known as "cutting vegetables on the chopping board." Visualize your hand as a knife, and slide the lateral edge (pinky-side) of the hand back and forth as if you are cutting vegetables on the edge of table with it. Practice this action 50 times, and then change to the other hand. Do this once or twice a day.

Frequent practice of this exercise can not only cure such symptoms as face flush and rapid heartbeat, but also relieve fatigue. It may also help to eliminate aches in the shoulders, head, back and groin area as well as numbness of the neck and spasmodic pain in the fingers, elbows and arms.

This method is effective, simple and time-saving, and especially useful for office workers who often sit in front of computers and students who have been holding books and pens for a long time. If they practice this method when feeling tired during work and study, it can help to relieve their fatigue.

Tianzong Point Helps with Hyperplasia of Mammary Glands

Hyperplasia of the mammary glands is a common disease among women. Its major feature is lateral or bilateral breast pain or lumps, and its incidence ranks first among all breast diseases. Recently the incidence of this disease has been rising year by year, with patients younger and younger. It is very common among women aged 25 to 45.

Periodic pain often happens, and at the beginning, diffusive swelling pain prevails, triggering an obvious sense of pain in the outer and central-upper part of the breast. Before the menstrual period the pain becomes more and more serious. After the menstrual period the pain subsides or disappears. However patients with a serious state of illness may suffer from continuous pain both before and after the menstrual period, with the scope of pain stretching from the breast to the armpit, shoulders, back and arms.

Hyperplasia of the mammary glands is called "lump in breast" in traditional Chinese medicine, because it is caused by the stagnation of energy and blood. It occurs when the liver is impaired by accumulated anger and the spleen is impaired by over-anxiety. Emotional change leads to disrupted energy and blood, and the stagnation of blood in the breast leads to pain.

In order to prevent and cure this hyperplasia, it is important to first regulate our meridians and acupoints. The Tianzong point is an important acupoint on the Small Intestine Meridian for curing female diseases. Frequent massaging of this acupoint can clear the meridians and acupoints, regulate vital energy, dissipate swelling, remove stasis, and prevent and cure various breast diseases.

To locate the Tianzong point, lie flat on your stomach. First find the depression at the center of the infraspinous fossa of the shoulder blade, and then the Tianzong point will be located at the upper one-third bend between the lower edge of the scapular

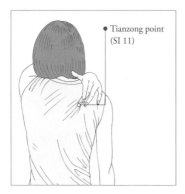

Tianzong point
(SI 11)

Massaging Tianzong Point Can Cure Breast Diseases

Sitting upright place your left hand on the center of the right shoulder, and reach downward to touch the Tianzong point with the tip of your middle finger. Massaging this acupoint frequently can clear meridians and acupoints, regulate vital energy, dissipate swelling, and prevent and cure various breast diseases.

spine and the inferior angle of the scapula. Or when sitting up straight in a chair, place your left hand on the center of the right shoulder. Press downward with the fingers, and the tip of the middle finger will touch the Tianzong point.

After accurately locating the acupoint, place your fingers near the Tianzong point for massaging. If you feel pain when your fingers touch a spot, this spot should be massaged and kneaded strongly. According to the feedback of most women who have suffered from breast diseases, they can very easily find this sore spot.

This spot is important because it is a "special-effect point" for curing acute and chronic mammitis and hyperplasia of the mammary glands. If the spot cannot be found it may simply indicate that your symptoms are relatively mild. In this case you can directly massage the Tianzong point. To massage use the techniques of "point-and-press" or tapping. Practice the above-mentioned action on this point for 15 to 20 minutes, once or twice a day.

Malar Rash, a Disease of the Small Intestine

Also called "chloasma" or "melisma," malar rash is a common phenomenon of skin pigmentation, mostly occurring on the faces of women, especially in the child-bearing period. It rarely happens to men.

If it remains over the long-term this pigmentation can have an effect on the image and self-esteem of some women. They often consult doctors, take various medicines and try different cosmetics, with no effect. However malar rashes can be cured effectively if the cause is understood properly and appropriate methods are employed.

The Small Intestine Meridian passes through the cheekbone, where malar rashes are mostly distributed. If the meridian at this place is not smooth or if the small intestine does not have a proper absorptive function, malar rashes naturally occur on the face. Regulating this meridian is the best method for preventing and curing malar rashes. In addition, the eyes may become yellow and the cheek swollen if the small intestine has a very poor function of absorption.

How to Exercise the Small Intestine Meridian

1. Stimulate the meridian from top to bottom with a hairbrush from the left and right shoulder blade. Then practice local stimulation on the meridian. Repeat 10 times.

2. Press and knead the rashes with the thumb pad, and make circles from the inside to the outside. Take care not to apply an extremely strong force, in case the skin should be hurt. Press and knead each spot where the pigmentation occurs for about one minute. Or after rubbing your palms together, placing them on the face, pressing and kneading the rashes clockwise. Apply a moderate force, and keep a moderate speed, so that the melanin can diffuse to all sides and become lighter.

Regulate Diet to Prevent and Eliminate Malar Rashes

1. Often eat foods containing Vitamin A, Vitamin C, protein and iron, for example spinach, carrot, egg, tomato, walnut,

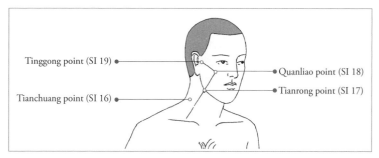

Tinggong point (SI 19)

Quanliao point (SI 18)

Tianrong point (SI 17)

Tianchuang point (SI 16)

Small Intestine Meridian's Path in the Head

This meridian passes through the cheekbone, and if it is disrupted here, or if the small intestine is not absorbing optimally, malar rashes may occur on the face.

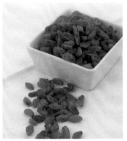

Raisins

raisin, beans, animal's liver and kidney.

2. Eat fewer dark-colored foods and drinks, for example strong tea, cola, coffee and chocolate. Eat more light-colored food, such as milk, egg, bean curd and fish, which can help to discharge the melanin in the body.

Yanglao Point Is a Magic Weapon

The small intestine has the functions of digesting food, absorbing nutritional substances and discharging waste. As a result of the functional aging of the small intestine, such phenomena as loss of appetite, reduction of food intake, and indigestion often happen to older people. These conditions can easily result in malnutrition, weak constitution, reduction of resistance, and the attack of such diseases as wind-cold, rheumatism and cold.

In addition, the degeneration of function often leads to abnormal excretion because the small intestine cannot normally eliminate waste. Under such circumstances the small intestine delivers to the large intestine the moisture that should have been delivered to the bladder. It also delivers to the bladder the waste that should have been delivered to the large intestine. Or else this waste builds up in the small intestine, giving rise to such problems as abdominal pain, diarrhea and difficult defecation, all of which are common among the elderly.

Old age is a time to enjoy leisure activities and family, and this is most achievable when one is not troubled by various diseases. There is a magic weapon that can help achieve this, not only preventing and curing these diseases but also prolonging life. The Yanglao point, an important acupoint on the Small Intestine Meridian, is reputed in TCM as "a magic weapon for old people to live a happy retired life."

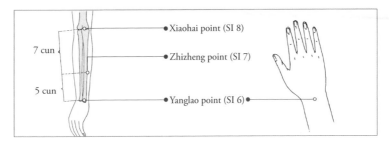

Locate the Yanglao Point

The benefits of the Yanglao point have long been recognized. According to *The Book of Rites*, a classic book of Chinese Confucianism, frequent massage as well as practicing acupuncture and moxibustion at the Yanglao point is as important to well-being as wearing insulated clothes to resist the cold and eating meat to fill the stomach.

The Yanglao point is located on the ulnar side at the back of the forearm, in the radial depression at the near end of the ulna capitulum. To locate the point, bend your elbow with the center of your palm facing your chest. Your Yanglao point will be located at the sutura (fibrous joint) on the same line with the highest point of the ulna capitulum. Or with the center of your palm facing downward, press the highest point of the ulna capitulum with another finger. Then change position to make the center of your palm face your chest, and the Yanglao point will be located at the sutura into which your finger slides.

Method

Pressing and kneading: Use the tip of the thumb to press, knead and rub the point for three to five minutes, once or twice a day; preferably from 1 to 3 p.m. At this time the energy and blood of the Small Intestine Meridian reach their prime so the best effect can be achieved from the action of pressing and kneading.

Moxibustion: If using moxa-cone moxibustion: 3 to 5 sections; moxa-stick moxibustion: 10–20 minutes.

Path of the Small Intestine Meridian

The Taiyang Small Intestine Meridian of Hand, abbreviated as "Small Intestine Meridian," starts from the Shaoze point on the outside of the tip of the little finger, connects with the Qiangu and Houxi points on its upper side, and goes along the ulnar side of the back of the hand. It passes the wrist and the rear edge of the outer arms, arrives at the elbow, goes to the rear of the shoulder joint, and then around the scapular region. The meridian crosses from the left and the right, and meets the Governing Vessel at the Dazhui point. Going forward it enters the supraclavicular fossa, goes into the body cavity and links with the heart. It then passes through the esophagus and diaphragm to arrive at the stomach. Moving downward it becomes part of the small intestine. Its

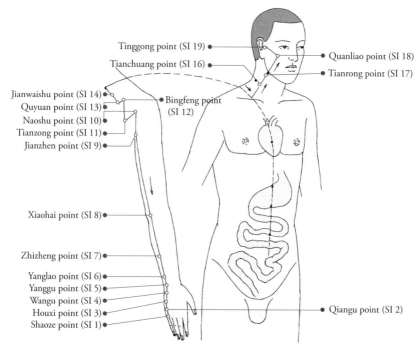

Tinggong point (SI 19)
Tianchuang point (SI 16)
Quanliao point (SI 18)
Tianrong point (SI 17)
Jianwaishu point (SI 14)
Quyuan point (SI 13)
Naoshu point (SI 10)
Tianzong point (SI 11)
Jianzhen point (SI 9)
Bingfeng point (SI 12)
Xiaohai point (SI 8)
Zhizheng point (SI 7)
Yanglao point (SI 6)
Yanggu point (SI 5)
Wangu point (SI 4)
Houxi point (SI 3)
Shaoze point (SI 1)
Qiangu point (SI 2)

Taiyang Small Intestine Meridian of Hand

branch separates from the cheek, goes upward and moves below the eyes. After moving on a diagonal to the lower edge of the eye socket, it passes the base of the nose, enters the inner eye corner (Jingming point), and connects with the Taiyang Bladder Meridian of Foot.

How to Exercise the Small Intestine Meridian

Arm swinging: This method is simple and convenient to practice. While standing swing both arms to and fro as far as you can, at a moderate speed. Do this exercise at least 100 times each round, once or twice a day. The first round should be between 9 to 11 a.m., and the second round between 1 to 3 p.m. If you only have time to do the exercise once a day it should be between 1 to 3 p.m.

This method not only exercises the muscles and reinforces stamina, but also smooths and clears all the meridians and collaterals that pass through the arms. It helps in relaxing tendons, activating collaterals, invigorating blood circulation and promoting muscle growth.

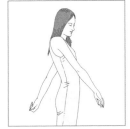

Swing arms to exercise Small Intestine Meridian.

Massaging: On the outside of the little finger, the Small Intestine Meridian is on the same line with the Shaoze and Qiangu points. Along this line we can massage the meridian from the tip to the base of the finger, so as to tonify the small intestine. Using this method frequently can cure such symptoms as deficiency-based cold, diuresis and enuresis. If you push from the base to the tip of the finger, you can purge the small intestine and cure such difficult urination symptoms as urodialysis. If the heat in the Heart Meridian is delivered to the small intestine, this method can also be used to remove heart-heat.

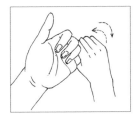

Massage to exercise Small Intestine Meridian.

119

Chapter Nine

Shen Time (3 p.m. to 5 p.m.)
Bladder Meridian in Its Prime

Shen Time (3 p.m. to 5 p.m.) is a golden period in the day, during which we have the most accurate judgment, strongest vigor and highest work efficiency. At Shen Time the Taiyang Bladder Meridian of Foot (Bladder Meridian), which connects the head and the feet, is in its prime; energy and blood flow past it, leaping up and down in this meridian.

At Shen Time we are very sober-minded, and therefore we can make judgments about important things at this time. In addition, we also have the strongest memory at Shen Time, and we can recite words and texts that are difficult to recite at other times. If students choose to review lessons at Shen Time, they will achieve an unexpected good result.

Shen Time is also a peak period for metabolism. One of the major organs for metabolism, the bladder is located in the lower abdomen. Just like a sewer pipe, the bladder is in charge of storing and discharging urine, expelling extra moisture from the body. At Shen Time, the Bladder Meridian works most efficiently, so at this time we can drink more water. Waste in the body can be transported to our bladder by the "sewer pipe," and expelled. As long as we ensure the smoothness of this transport system at any moment, the entire process of metabolism will be optimal. This can prevent and cure many diseases and eliminate many health-related hazards.

Maintain Healthy Urination by Replenishing Water

According to *Yellow Emperor's Inner Canon*, the bladder functions like the local official in charge of water. It is in charge of regulation through the storage and excretion of urine. Only after having been collected in the bladder can urine be expelled from the body. In order to maintain healthy urination, we must drink more water. This dilutes the blood, promotes food digestion, and maintains the skin, beauty and youth. It also relaxes the bowels, promotes diuresis and boosts metabolism.

When there is no flowing water to wash out the bladder, just like in a sewer, waste will back up and give off odor. Only after having been washed out frequently can the wastes in the bladder be smoothly expelled from the body, along with water and other liquids. In this way wastes and toxins can be removed in a timely manner, leaving us to feel comfortable and refreshed all over.

It is important to modify our water drinking habits according to the clock. From 8 to 10 a.m., we begin work or movement, and therefore also begin perspiring. Drinking water at this time can replenish the lost water in the body. We should drink more water in the afternoon, especially at Shen Time, when the Bladder Meridian is in its prime. At this time it has the most energy and blood and the strongest capacity for action. In addition, the food we have

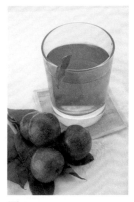

Water

eaten for lunch arrives at the bladder then, after due digestion and absorption.

Replenishing water at this time increases the flow in the bladder, quickly clearing waste from the body. If we cannot replenish water at this time, waste accumulates and remains in the bladder, thus giving rise to urination problems and urocystitis, and possible even bladder stones and cancer. Therefore drinking more water, especially at Shen Time, is extremely important for one's health. One should also drink water one hour before sleep. Since the viscosity of the blood reaches a high degree before sleep, drinking water at this time can dilute blood, expand blood vessels and benefit the body.

Improve Memory by Massaging Xinshu Point

Memory relates to brain activity, and the brain is indirectly regulated and controlled by the Bladder Meridian. Among the twelve main meridians, the Bladder Meridian has the most sufficient yang energy. Known as a "small sun" in the human body, the Bladder Meridian indirectly improves brain function by regulating the energy and blood of the kidney.

Sufficient energy and blood in the brain can ensure quick thinking, precise judgment and effective memory. On the contrary, if the kidneys are weak, the Bladder Meridian is unable to allocate enough energy and blood to the brain, so that it reacts slowly and memory declines considerably. This is a universal phenomenon among people between 40 and 50 years old. This is because at this age, various functions of the body decline, and the vital energy in the kidneys becomes insufficient. The deficiency of energy and blood brings about the weaker reaction of the brain and the decline of memory.

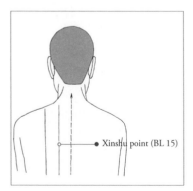
Xinshu point (BL 15)

Massaging Xinshu point can improve memory.

One need not worry too much about the decline of memory because there are methods for improvement. Massaging the Xinshu point can improve memory. As a part of the Taiyang Bladder Meridian of Foot, this important acupoint is located in the back, about the width of two fingers (or about 1.5 cun) below the spinous process of the fifth thoracic vertebra, both on the left and the right side. Massaging this acupoint at Shen Time produces the best results.

Sleepiness at Shen Time Indicates Yang Deficiency

According to traditional Chinese medicine, if yang energy remains insufficient in the body, or if vital energy and blood are weak, we become listless and drowsy. This is opposite to how we should feel at Shen Time: alive, energetic and quick-minded.

As the main meridian with the most yang energy, the Bladder Meridian runs through nearly the whole human body from top to bottom. The yang energy in the body is chiefly transported by this meridian. In addition, the Bladder Meridian has a relationship of mutual reliance and manifestation with the Kidney Meridian. Their energy and blood, as well as their functions, are interconnected. The yang energy in the kidneys is jointly regulated by these two meridians.

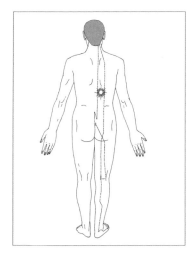

Our mental state has something to do with the heart, brain and kidneys. The heart is in charge of spirit and will, but it needs to be supported by the brain and kidneys. In the final

Bladder Meridian, Known as the "Small Sun" of the Body
As the meridian with the most sufficient yang energy among the twelve main meridians, the Bladder Meridian transports most of the yang energy in the body.

analysis the Bladder Meridian is closely related to mental state. If the yang energy in the Bladder Meridian is sufficient and the meridian is smooth, we will feel vigorous and energetic. However if the yang energy is weak and the meridian is not smooth, we will become tired, listless and sleepy. In particular feeling sleepy at Shen Time (when the Bladder Meridian is in its prime) surely indicates yang deficiency in the body.

Solution

1. Tap along the circulatory route of the Bladder Meridian in the back and legs with your fist or a small hammer (TCM medical instrument). Move first from bottom to top, then from top to bottom. This method can promote circulation of energy and blood in the Bladder Meridian, relax tendons and activate collaterals.

2. Massage the Yongquan point at the sole of the feet. This method can promote yang energy all over the body and strengthen kidney functions.

Important Cause of Rheumatic Arthritis

In *Yellow Emperor's Inner Canon*, wind, coldness and dampness are jointly called "rheumatism." Since rheumatism mostly involves joints and triggers pain, the modern phrase "rheumatic arthritis" is applied. Medically, rheumatic arthritis is a common acute or chronic inflammation of connective tissue.

Most patients have such symptoms as light or moderate fever and joint pain. The joints involved include the knee, ankle, shoulder and wrist, and the pain can be transferred from one joint to another. The achy parts tend to turn red, swollen and scorching hot, with repeated attacks of pain. As an allergic disease, it is one of the major manifestations of rheumatic fever.

Rheumatic arthritis is an obstinate disease. Although there are many causes of this disease, in the final analysis it is caused by injury to meridians and collaterals in the body. Running from head to feet, the Bladder Meridian serves as the "warehouse" for yang energy, continually transporting yang energy to the body to ensure the normal operation of various "departments." Once a problem happens to the Bladder Meridian, yin and yang lose their balance, and one can contract rheumatism if any pathogen invades at this time.

Damage to the Bladder Meridian, which passes through such parts as the feet, ankles, knees and shoulders, results in disrupted blood circulation in the body. Most nutrition is transported along with blood, and if blood circulation is not smooth, some parts of the body do not receive sufficient nutrition. This can cause diseases of local tissues to occur, e.g. muscular atrophy and arthritis. Disrupted blood flow also leads to turbid phlegm and blood stasis, which can easily accumulate at some joints and trigger inflammation. This is also why rheumatic arthritis cannot be cured radically.

Preventing Rheumatism by Regulating Bladder Meridian

To regulate the Bladder Meridian, frequent tapping along the route of the meridian on the back is recommended, as is vigorous massage of sore parts. This method can relax tendons, activate collaterals and dissipate blood stasis. As the meridian with the most sufficient yang energy among the twelve main meridians, the Bladder Meridian transports most of the yang energy in the body.

Massaging rheumatic parts can improve their blood circulation.

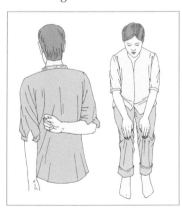

Tap along the route of the meridian on the back to remove dampness and massage rheumatic parts to improve blood circulation.

Improve Eye Health by Kneading Tianzhu Point

As can be seen from the circulatory route diagram of the Bladder Meridian, it has an extremely long route, moving from head to feet, and passing through many acupoints of different sizes. These acupoints have their respective special roles, and regulating them can prevent and cure many diseases.

The Tianzhu point is an important acupoint on the Bladder Meridian. It plays a role in refreshing us, improving our eyesight and relieving visual fatigue. For people who need to use their eyes for a long time, massaging this acupoint can prevent their eyesight from declining.

The Tianzhu point is located in the middle of the back of the neck, at the recession of the upper edge of the two vertical muscles, and about 2 cm beside the middle of the rear hairline.

How to Massage the Tianzhu Point

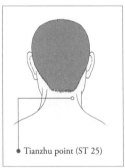

Tianzhu point (ST 25)

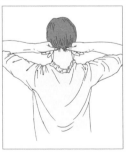

1. Press the Tianzhu point on both sides with due force with your thumb, exhaling with mouth wide open at the same time. Repeat this action 5 times.

2. Press this acupoint with the pad of your thumb, using a strong force. Be sure to raise your jaw and stretch your head backward. After pressing each acupoint for 5 seconds, suddenly increase the pressure and then relax. Repeat 5 to 10 times.

3. After rubbing both hands together to produce heat, cross your fingers behind your neck at the base of your head. Place the center of the palms on the left and right Tianzhu point in your neck, and press downward for 3 to 5 minutes. Repeat 3 times.

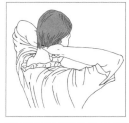

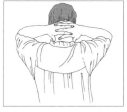

With increased use of the eyes at close range for a long time (e.g. reading, writing, using the computer), more and more people have become near-sighted. Frequent massaging of the Tianzhu point is helpful for recovering eyesight, as well as preventing near-sightedness and keeping it from worsening. This method is also suitable for middle-aged and older people, who are most afflicted by eye problems. Massaging the Tianzhu point can not only improve eyesight and restore consciousness, but also slow down the blurring of an image. In addition to massaging this point, we should often do eye exercises, gaze at green plants, look into the distance, and eat more vitamin-containing vegetables and fruits.

How to Exercise the Bladder Meridian

Abbreviated as the Bladder Meridian, the Taiyang Bladder Meridian of Foot starts from the Jingming point at the inner eye corner, and ends at the Zhiyin point on the outer edge of the little toe. It is divided into two branches at the head. One branch separates from the Baihui point at the top of the head, and extends toward the upper corner of the ear. The other branch goes from the top of the head downward (to the Naohu point), enters the cranium and links with the brain, and then returns and goes downward to the Tianzhu point at the back of neck.

The two branches go downward and meet each other at the Dazhui point. From here this meridian is again divided into two branches (left and right). One branch starts from the Dazhui point in the inner shoulder, presses the spine from both sides, and travels along a route about 1.5 cun away from the dorsal line. It goes down

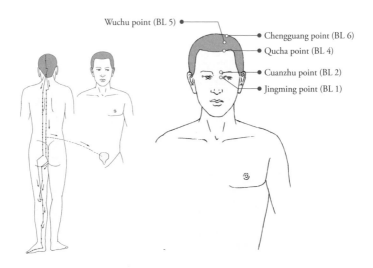

Wuchu point (BL 5)
Chengguang point (BL 6)
Qucha point (BL 4)
Cuanzhu point (BL 2)
Jingming point (BL 1)

Taiyang Bladder Meridian of Foot (Part)

to the waist, enters the muscle beside the spine, and links with the kidney. Continuing downward, it becomes a part of bladder, and then separates from the waist and goes down once more, again pressing the spine from both sides. It communicates with the hip, passes the rear of the leg, and enters the popliteal fossa.

The other branch goes downward from the inner shoulder, passes through it, and then descends along a route about 3 cun away from the dorsal line, It passes through the hip, goes past the Huantiao point of the hip joint, downward along the rear of the outer leg, and meets at the popliteal fossa. Continuing downward it runs through the musculus gastrocnemius, goes past the Kunlun point at the back of the outer ankle, turns and goes forward at the heel. Passing the outer dorsum of foot, it arrives at the Zhiyin point on the outer edge of the little toe, and connects with the Shaoyin Kidney Meridian of Foot.

As mentioned previously the Bladder Meridian has the most sufficient yang energy among all meridians in the human body, and therefore, it is a very important meridian. Now we will

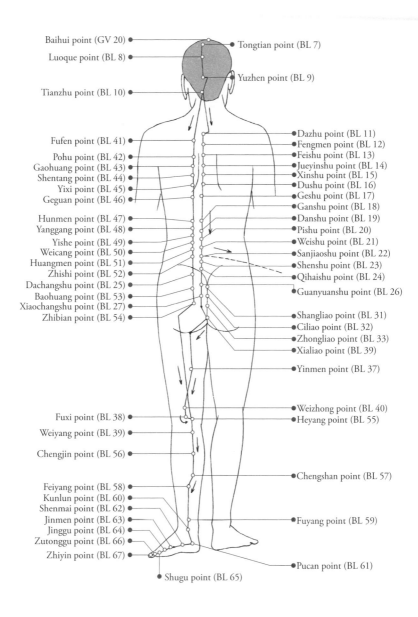

Baihui point (GV 20)
Luoque point (BL 8)
Tongtian point (BL 7)
Yuzhen point (BL 9)
Tianzhu point (BL 10)

Fufen point (BL 41)
Pohu point (BL 42)
Gaohuang point (BL 43)
Shentang point (BL 44)
Yixi point (BL 45)
Geguan point (BL 46)
Hunmen point (BL 47)
Yanggang point (BL 48)
Yishe point (BL 49)
Weicang point (BL 50)
Huangmen point (BL 51)
Zhishi point (BL 52)
Dachangshu point (BL 25)
Baohuang point (BL 53)
Xiaochangshu point (BL 27)
Zhibian point (BL 54)

Dazhu point (BL 11)
Fengmen point (BL 12)
Feishu point (BL 13)
Jueyinshu point (BL 14)
Xinshu point (BL 15)
Dushu point (BL 16)
Geshu point (BL 17)
Ganshu point (BL 18)
Danshu point (BL 19)
Pishu point (BL 20)
Weishu point (BL 21)
Sanjiaoshu point (BL 22)
Shenshu point (BL 23)
Qihaishu point (BL 24)
Guanyuanshu point (BL 26)

Shangliao point (BL 31)
Ciliao point (BL 32)
Zhongliao point (BL 33)
Xialiao point (BL 39)

Yinmen point (BL 37)

Weizhong point (BL 40)
Heyang point (BL 55)

Fuxi point (BL 38)
Weiyang point (BL 39)
Chengjin point (BL 56)

Chengshan point (BL 57)

Feiyang point (BL 58)
Kunlun point (BL 60)
Shenmai point (BL 62)
Jinmen point (BL 63)
Jinggu point (BL 64)
Zutonggu point (BL 66)
Zhiyin point (BL 67)

Fuyang point (BL 59)

Pucan point (BL 61)

Shugu point (BL 65)

Taiyang Bladder Meridian of Foot (Part)

learn how to maintain and exercise this meridian, especially the sections in our back and legs.

Back

The back of the body is not only the major area passed by the Bladder Meridian, but also a refuge for our internal organs. Therefore nourishing the Bladder Meridian means protecting our internal organs. It is very important to reinforce the maintenance of this section. The best exercise method is tapping the back from top to bottom with the hand or a healthcare hammer along the route of the Bladder Meridian, 10 to 15 minutes each time.

Legs

The Bladder Meridian has a vital acupoint in the legs: the Weizhong point. This acupoint is located at the midpoint of the popliteal crease behind the knee, and between the tendon of the biceps femoris and the tendon of the semitendinosus. The damp and hot moisture of the Bladder Meridian gathers here. Frequently stimulating this acupoint can balance yin and yang energy. It can be exercised by using the following methods, preferably at Shen Time because the best effect can be achieved at this time.

1. Press the Weizhong point with the tip of the thumb, with a force that produces a faint ache. Press and release continuously, 10 to 20 times.

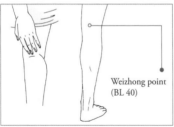

Weizhong point
(BL 40)

Massage Weizhong point to balance yin and yang.

2. After rubbing hands together vigorously, rub this acupoint with the palmar surfaces of both hands, back and forth and up and down. Do this 30 times.

Chapter Ten

You Time (5 p.m. to 7 p.m.)
Kidney Meridian in Its Prime

At You Time (5 p.m. to 7 p.m.), the sun sets in the west, with yang energy on the earth slowly subsiding and yin energy gradually growing. At this time the Shaoyin Kidney Meridian of Foot (Kidney Meridian) is at work, with energy and blood flowing past it, and the vital essence of the body stored in the kidneys.

The kidneys are the origin of congenital constitution, the essence with which we are born. Furthermore, according to TCM, the kidneys govern bones and generate marrow, which communicates with the brain. Therefore the kidneys are closely related to intelligence and thinking ability. The kidneys play a decisive role in genius and heredity in humans.

The kidneys have the function of storing vital essence. Congenital vital essence inherited from our parents is generally stored in the kidneys; acquired vital essence—influenced by diet, environment and other factors from birth onward—is also stored in the kidneys in addition to being supplied to the internal organs.

If the vital essence in our kidneys is sufficient, then our bones, teeth and hair can grow properly. In addition, the vital essence in our kidneys can also generate a substance called the "heavenly tenth," which can promote the maturity of reproductive function, influencing the generation of semen and menses. Insufficient vital essence in the kidneys affects bones and hearing.

The hypofunction of the kidneys in storing vital essence not only slows down development in children, but also affects the tissues and functions maintained by vital essence.

The kidneys also regulate the metabolic function of body fluids. Body fluids are evenly transported to and distributed in various parts of the human body only when the physiological function of the kidneys is normal. They ensure that redundant moisture is normally discharged from the body after having been transformed into urine. The function of the bladder is also controlled by the kidneys. If the kidneys have a low function in controlling the metabolism of body fluids, it causes such problems as edema, hypofunction of the bladder, urodynia, and other urination disorders including problems with frequency.

In addition, the kidneys can reinforce the physiological function of the lungs, and help maintain regular breathing movement.

Since the kidneys are vital for the human body, we must take good care of them in our daily life. You Time is the most suitable time during the day for nourishing the kidneys. This is because our Kidney Meridian is in its prime, the energy and blood in this meridian is the most sufficient, and it has the strongest ability to take in and store vital essence at this time.

The kidneys are associated with winter, and so among the four seasons, winter is the most suitable one for tonifying the kidneys. Winter is the season when living things hide themselves for recuperation. In winter the yang energy on the earth hides itself deeply and the cold yin energy prevails. The kidneys collect Shaoyin energy in the body so as to live through the long and cold winter.

In winter you should go to bed earlier and get up later, keep out of the cold and try to stay in warm places, and avoid perspiring too much. This will protect vital energy from damage. If we violate the law of collection in winter, the Shaoyin energy in our body cannot be hidden away, the ability of the kidneys to distinguish between essence and waste will decline, and the kidneys will be impaired, thus doing harm to our health.

Winter generates cold, which corresponds with moisture. In turn moisture generates saltiness, which enters the kidneys. Saltiness can create kidney energy, which can generate marrow. Enriched marrow nourishes the liver. Eating a moderate amount of salty food can benefit the kidneys; however eating too much salty food considerably undermines vigor. The kidneys show preference for black food. Therefore eating more black food, for example black fungus, black sesame, walnut, black bean porridge and black rice porridge, will help to tonify the kidneys.

Women Also Vulnerable to Kidney Deficiency

Many people mistakenly believe that deficiency of the kidneys caused by insufficient kidney essence happens to males only, and never to females. As a matter of fact, women are also vulnerable to this deficiency, with such symptoms as lifeless and dull hair, menstrual disorder, pale face and prematurely graying hair.

As we have learned the kidneys are a place where the vital essence of the body is stored. All of the body's essence, energy and spirit come from the kidneys. Some women have a weak physical constitution, suffer often from minor diseases, and do not pay attention to nutrition. Therefore they do not have enough yang energy in their body or vital essence in their kidneys, and suffer from kidney deficiency.

Work pressure is also a cause of this deficiency. Many women nowadays face a greater and greater workload, and often work overtime. Moreover they do not pay enough attention to rest. Therefore they consume too much vital essence, and their kidneys are overburdened by the duty of trying to keep up with supplying vital essence to their bodies. In the long run, deficiency of the kidneys results.

This phenomenon often happens to women during breast-feeding. Mothers have to face the challenges of supplying enough nutrition to their babies and looking after them continually. In particular their nights may be disrupted by children who often cry and scream. As a result it is very difficult for them to take care of their own bodies, which may cause kidney deficiency.

In addition, a poor work environment may also negatively influence the health of the kidneys. If one works in an unventilated air-conditioned environment for a long time, the hazardous substances in the air (carbon dioxide, toxins, dust, etc.) may impair the immune function of the internal organs including the kidneys. This can result in nephritis in the long run. Once our kidneys cannot store enough vital essence, deficiency of the kidneys occurs.

Kidney deficiency in women can be classified into yin deficiency and yang deficiency. Women suffering from yin deficiency of the kidneys are particularly adverse to cold; catch colds easily; remain low-spirited all day; have dry, dark and lusterless skin; exhibit black eyes and a face covered with chloasma; experience hair loss; or become infertile and devoid of sexual desire. Women suffering from yang deficiency feel soreness and weakness in their waist and knees; often suffer from dizziness and tinnitus; experience heat in the palm and sole; suffer from constipation; or have such symptoms as the postponement of the menstrual period, scanty menstruation and amenorrhea.

Therefore women suffering from kidney deficiency must determine whether they have yin or yang deficiency before nourishing their kidneys. It is best to consult an experienced doctor of traditional Chinese medicine for a diagnosis. They should maintain good indoor air ventilation, avoid staying in an air-conditioned environment for a long time, drink more water, and avoid overwork. They should also pay special attention to their diet.

Women suffering from yin deficiency of the kidneys can

often eat such yin-nourishing food as Chinese wolfberry, lotus seed, lily bulb, agaric, mulberry, lotus root, fish, black sesame and walnut. Women suffering from yang deficiency can eat such yang-nourishing food as beef, cinnamon, longan, Chinese leek, Chinese yam and mutton. Women suffering from kidney deficiency should eat less raw, cold and pungent food, such as water chestnut, persimmon, raw carrot or cucumber, watermelon, melon, onion, chili, leaf mustard, pepper, mint, liquor and tobacco, which may aggravate the state of their illness.

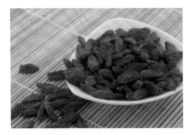
Chinese Wolfberry

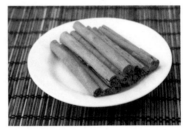
Cinnamon

Elderly Can Nourish Kidneys through Footbaths

There is an old Chinese saying that bathing the feet in hot water is more beneficial than eating ginseng. TCM also holds that we should bathe our feet in all four seasons, and that bathing the feet in different seasons can produce different effects. The most crucial aspect of health preservation for the elderly is nourishing the kidneys, and bathing the feet is one of the best ways to

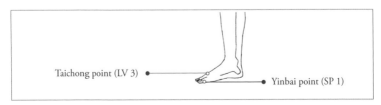

Taichong point (LV 3)

Yinbai point (SP 1)

Taichong and Yinbai Points

accomplish this.

As one reaches old age, all body functions are on the decline. The most obvious expression is the deficiency and failure of the kidneys. People with unhealthy kidneys have such symptoms as hair loss, tinnitus, deafness, dizziness, loose teeth, indigestion, constipation, insomnia and numb joints. Bathing the feet can stimulate the Taichong, Yinbai, Taixi and Yongquan points in the feet as well as various acupoints below the ankle. This helps in nourishing vital energy, regulating internal organs, clearing meridians, promoting metabolism and slowing down senility, and helping to improve and cure other symptoms attributed to unhealthy kidneys in the elderly.

Ways of Footbaths

Although bathing the feet can help prolong life, we must use an appropriate method. In a footbath basin, add water at a temperature that makes your feet feel warm. Pour enough water into the basin so that the water has just immersed your entire foot. Soak your feet in the basin for five to ten minutes. Then repeatedly rub and knead the top, sole and toes of your feet with your hands.

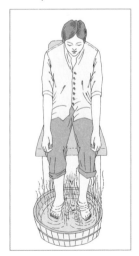

Bathing feet is one of the best ways to nourish kidneys.

You should locate important acupoints in your feet (e.g. Yongquan, Taixi, Taichong, Yinbai and Zhaohai points), then rub and knead them strongly. If the water becomes cold, add more hot water, and continue to rub and knead your feet. After finishing the footbath, you can rub and knead your feet with a dry towel for another 20 to 30 minutes. It is best for your health if you bathe your feet at night, and go to bed 30 minutes afterward. This is most helpful for the generation of yang energy.

Benefits of Footbaths

1. Regulating kidney energy: Frequent bathing of the feet can help to expand blood vessels, promote blood circulation in the feet, clear tendons and muscles, and help in nourishing the kidneys and liver.

2. Preventing cold: Footbaths can prevent cold and bring down fever. When both feet are immersed in hot water, their blood vessels begin to expand. This results in the reflective expansion of blood vessels all over the body, and the smooth and vigorous flow of blood. This can also reinforce the function of the sweat glands, so that heat can be dissipated through the evaporation of perspiration.

3. Reducing blood pressure: While bathing our feet, we can massage the Yongquan point and press the Taichong point (located in the outer dorsum of the foot behind the hallux toe), which can help reduce blood pressure.

4. Curing rheumatism: Bathing the feet can promote smooth blood circulation in aching parts, thus removing blood stasis and relieving pain.

5. Curing headache: Footbaths help to dilate the blood vessels in the feet, so that the blood flows from the head to the feet. This can reduce cerebral congestion and relieve headache.

How to Exercise the Kidney Meridian

The kidneys are the origin of congenital constitution, or inherited health, and a place for storing vital essence. Our essence, energy and spirit stem from our kidneys, which exert their function through regulation of the Kidney Meridian. Therefore exercising the Kidney Meridian can protect and nourish our kidneys.

The Shaoyin Kidney Meridian of Foot starts from the lower little toe, goes obliquely toward the sole of the foot, and out from the lower tuberosity of the tarsal navicular bone. Moving upward along the rear inner ankle to the shin side of the lower leg (with its branch entering the heel), it emerges from the shin side of the popliteal fossa. Traveling upward to the rear side of the inner thigh, it passes the spine, becomes part of the kidneys and links with the bladder. Its trunk (direct-movement meridian) goes upward from the kidneys, passes the liver and diaphragm, and enters the lungs. Moving along the throat, it presses the root of tongue from both sides. A branch separates from the lungs, connects with the heart, flows in the chest, and links with the Jueyin Pericardium Meridian of Hand.

The main method for exercising the Kidney Meridian is massaging this meridian where it travels in the stomach and massaging acupoints on the soles.

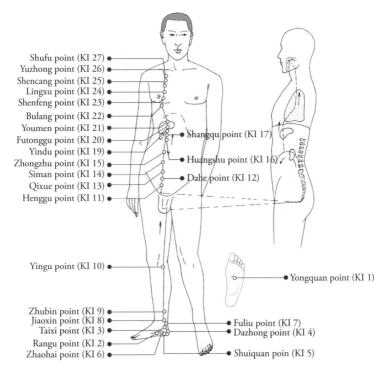

Shufu point (KI 27)
Yuzhong point (KI 26)
Shencang point (KI 25)
Lingxu point (KI 24)
Shenfeng point (KI 23)
Bulang point (KI 22)
Youmen point (KI 21)
Futonggu point (KI 20)
Yindu point (KI 19)
Zhongzhu point (KI 15)
Siman point (KI 14)
Qixue point (KI 13)
Henggu point (KI 11)

Shangqu point (KI 17)
Huangshu point (KI 16)
Dahe point (KI 12)

Yingu point (KI 10)

Yongquan point (KI 1)

Zhubin point (KI 9)
Jiaoxin point (KI 8)
Taixi point (KI 3)
Rangu point (KI 2)
Zhaohai point (KI 6)

Fuliu point (KI 7)
Dazhong point (KI 4)

Shuiquan poin (KI 5)

Shaoyin Kidney Meridian of Foot

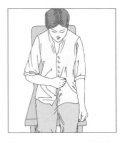

Do the massage of Kidney Meridian in the abdomen.

Sitting in a chair, use your palm or clench your hand into a fist. Press and knead up and down from heart to abdomen, 5 to 10 minutes a time. Exercise once a day, preferably at You Time. This method can effectively clear the Kidney Meridian in the chest and abdomen, and help to maintain smooth energy and blood.

The Kidney Meridian has three important acupoints in the feet: Yongquan, Zhaohai and Taixi.

The Yongquan point is located in the front third of the sole of the foot, at the depression when the toes are bent. Sit with crossed legs, and massage with both hands or press the Yongquan point on both sides with the tip of a bent finger, preferably with a force that can produce an aching and swelling feeling, for 50 to 100 times each round. If you persist in doing this year round, you can naturally reinforce the function of the kidneys.

The Zhaohai point is located at the depression under the tip of the inner condyle. The Taixi point is located at the depression slightly in the upper part of the rear of the tip of the inner condyle. These two acupoints can be pressed with a fingertip. After accurately locating the acupoints, press each one for about three minutes with the finger pad, using a slight force. Or press and knead the acupoints on both feet at the same time using your hands. Frequently massaging these two acupoints can regulate

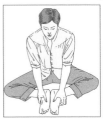

Massage the Yongquan point.

kidney energy and prevent such kidney diseases as nephritis and kidney deficiency. It can also relieve and cure such symptoms as neurasthenia, epilepsy, irregular menstruation, toothache, swelling and pain of the throat, asthma, bronchitis, cold hands and feet, arthritis and hand rheumatalgia.

Chapter Eleven

Xu Time (7 p.m. to 9 p.m.)
Pericardium Meridian in Its Prime

At Xu Time (7 p.m. to 9 p.m.) night falls gradually, the moon slowly rises, and yin energy reaches its peak in the heavens and on earth. With yang energy vanishing slowly, we quiet down after the busy day.

We all know that the heart is a very important yet sometimes fragile organ. If emotions (including pleasure, anger, sorrow and joy) are too strong, or moods change too quickly, it can impair the heart. A thin membrane wrapping the heart, the pericardium plays an important role in protecting it. Between the pericardium and the wall of the heart there is serous fluid, which can lubricate the heart muscle. This prevents the heart from being impaired due to friction with the thoracic cavity as it pumps blood. The Jueyin Pericardium Meridian of Hand (Pericardium Meridian) connects the pericardium and heart, and functions optimally at Xu Time.

As we have seen, *Yellow Emperor's Inner Canon* assigns a role to each of the major organs, and the pericardium is like an official who serves the emperor. It endures all emotions first. For example when we are angry, the emotion of anger is initially delivered to the pericardium through the Pericardium Meridian, so that the pericardium experiences the emotion first, before being delivered to the heart.

The pericardium not only reacts to emotions such as joy

and anger, but it also suffers pathological factors on behalf of the heart. When a pathogen invades, the pericardium serves as the first barrier. In this way the heart sustains much less injury.

However the pericardium is quite vulnerable to emotion, and tends to be suffocated or separate due to the change of our moods. Therefore we should protect our pericardium as an initial line of defense in protecting our heart, keeping it safe and sound.

Nourish Heart and Stomach Shortly after Supper

People with a strong heart function also have a strong function of the spleen and stomach. On the contrary, poor function of the spleen and stomach affects the blood supply of the heart. Therefore we can protect the heart by taking good care of the spleen and stomach.

Xu Time is a golden occasion for nourishing the heart and stomach, coming directly after supper. Doing vigorous exercises after supper is not beneficial to the health of our spleen and kidneys. It is best to do more gentle exercises half an hour after eating.

There is an old saying that taking a walk after a meal prolongs life. Many people, especially older people, often go out for a walk after eating because they believe this can promote digestion and improve their health. The truth is the opposite. After a meal some food still remains in the esophagus. So if we move about immediately, the food may be jammed in its path, thus resulting

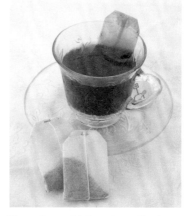

Please do not drink tea immediately after meal.

in obstruction. In addition, blood flows to the stomach at this time. Walking would scatter our energy and blood, thus affecting digestion and impairing the health of the spleen and stomach.

Some people have developed a habit of drinking tea immediately after meal, because they believe this can not only rinse the mouth but also promote digestion. This common practice is also harmful to the health.

If we drink tea immediately after a meal, a lot of water enters the stomach, diluting the digestive juice secreted by our kidneys. This prevents food from being digested in the stomach. In addition, tea contains a lot of tannic acid. If we drink tea immediately after a meal, the protein still remaining in the stomach will become an indigestible solid in combination with tannic acid, thus affecting its digestion and absorption.

More importantly, tea prevents the body from absorbing iron. For example if we drink tea brewed with 15 grams of dry tea after a meal, the absorption of iron from the food would decrease by 50%. In the long run this practice affects digestive function, and may even result in iron-deficiency anemia. Therefore drinking tea immediately after a meal is taboo in terms of health preservation.

After a meal, listening to music is recommended. According to *Protection of Vital Essence for Longevity*, a masterpiece written by an imperial doctor in the 17th century during the Ming dynasty, "The spleen is fond of music. On hearing music, the spleen would move to grind food." Taoist theory also holds that listening to music after a meal can promote digestion.

In terms of modern medical theory, listening to music (especially soft, light and lively music) can be used as a benign stimulation to regulate the digestive and absorptive function of the body through the central nervous system. Therefore we can enjoy music after a meal to relax ourselves and promote digestion. Other recommended activities include appreciating distant scenery, watching television, and having a chat. It is best to wait to take a walk half an hour after a meal.

Sit with Crossed Legs to Replenish Vital Energy

"Both the spirit and will of people are stored in the heart and generated by the heart," as we learn in *Yellow Emperor's Inner Canon*. Sitting with crossed legs can benefit the heart by soothing the mind and soul, and replenishing vital energy.

After working strenuously for the entire day, people are advised to quiet down, sit with crossed legs, and close their eyes meditatively. This is a good method for setting the mind at rest. It also helps people to relax themselves physically and mentally, relieving their fatigue and increasing their work efficiency.

The method is simple. First sit with crossed legs in a quiet environment. Put both palms face down on the knees, or together in a "prayer position" in front of your chest. Close both eyes lightly. Relax yourself both physically and mentally. Keep calm and hold your breath, getting rid of all distracting thoughts. Use abdominal breathing, inhaling through the nose, and lowering the thoracic diaphragm. In the way the internal organs are squeezed downward, so that your belly rises instead of your chest. Upon exhalation the diaphragm rises, so that you can breathe deeply. In short you should inhale deeply and exhale slowly.

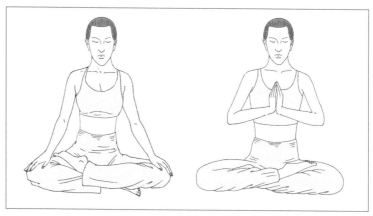

Sit with crossed legs and bent knees. Use the method of abdominal respiration.

This method can increase air throughput and reduce breathing frequency. Preferably it should be done at Xu Time, half an hour after supper. At this time the Pericardium Meridian is in its prime, so a better effect is achieved. Practice this about 15 minutes a day. Afterward you will feel comfortable both physically and mentally, and a regular practice over the long term will yield a more obvious effect.

Breast Disease Closely Related to Pericardium Meridian

In recent years the incidence of breast cancers has been higher and higher. According to data from the World Health Organization, there are well over one million new cases of breast cancer and a half million people die from this disease every year worldwide. However we are still extremely short of preventive and protective consciousness for this high-incidence disease. Moreover not only females but also males have become afflicted, and it is more difficult to radically cure in men. Breast disease has become a major threat to the health.

Is there any way to prevent incidence from growing? We should first get to know the causes. When meridians do not operate smoothly, this has a close relationship with the occurrence of hyperplasia of the mammary glands, breast nodules and even breast cancer. The Pericardium Meridian is an important meridian passing the outer breast. Any damage to the breast would be expressed through this meridian. Since breast disease is mostly related to this meridian, we can take a step toward prevention by regulating our Pericardium Meridian.

Putting aside other issues, the occurrence of breast disease can also have something to do with the change of moods. As we have learned the change of moods afflicts the pericardium first before being conducted to the heart. The Pericardium Meridian is the direct connection between the heart and pericardium.

If this meridian is not smooth, moods cannot be dispersed in a timely manner, thus resulting in depression. Anger, depression, gloominess and stasis of energy and blood can lead to breast disease. Therefore we should take good care of the Pericardium Meridian, as well as taking care not to get angry at trivial matters in daily life. Maintaining a healthy and happy state of mind is beneficial to breast health.

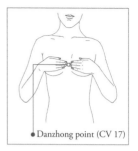

Danzhong point (CV 17)

Massage the Danzhong point.

The Danzhong point is an important acupoint on the Pericardium Meridian. Located at the midpoint between the nipples, it belongs to the Conception Vessel (*Ren Mai*), and lies close to the breast. It is known as one of the most important acupoints for gynecology and it is the best acupoint for preventing and curing diseases related to the mammary gland system. Frequently massaging the Danzhong point can relieve hyperplasia of the mammary glands.

We can self-massage this point using the techniques of kneading and pushing. Knead, using the tip of the middle finger, for about two minutes a time. Push from bottom to top, along the anterior median line from the Danzhong point, using the pads of the thumbs of both hands. Move slowly and evenly for about two minutes.

Kneading and pushing can regulate the Conception Vessel and Vital Vessel (*Chong Mai*), tonify vital energy and blood, and soothe the liver. It can also stimulate menstrual flow, prevent and cure such diseases as hyperplasia of the mammary glands, mammitis, chest pain and asthma, and effectively cure maldevelopment of the breast, mammary ptosis and scanty postnatal milk.

It is important to pay sufficient attention to breast healthcare. In our daily life, we should not only develop healthy living habits and maintain an optimistic state of mind, but also regulate our own meridians, thus staying far away from breast disease.

How to Exercise the Pericardium Meridian

At Xu Time (7 p.m. to 9 p.m.) the Pericardium Meridian is in its prime, with vital energy and blood flowing past the pericardium. Since the Pericardium Meridian connects the pericardium and heart, it is important to maintain its smooth passage, which will in turn protect the heart.

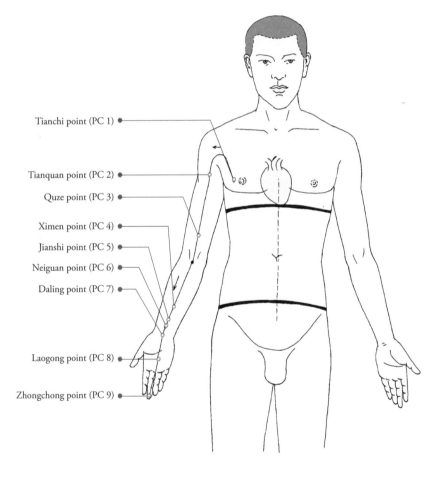

Tianchi point (PC 1)

Tianquan point (PC 2)

Quze point (PC 3)

Ximen point (PC 4)

Jianshi point (PC 5)

Neiguan point (PC 6)

Daling point (PC 7)

Laogong point (PC 8)

Zhongchong point (PC 9)

Jueyin Pericardium Meridian of Hand

From 7 p.m. to 8 p.m. most people have their supper. After a busy and tiring day, this is the time for relaxation. However, although not widely known, this is also the best time for protecting and nourishing the heart. While watching television, chatting or surfing the Internet, we can use our hands to do something beneficial to our health: pressing and kneading the Pericardium Meridian.

Abbreviated as the Pericardium Meridian, the Jueyin Pericardium Meridian of Hand passes the inner arm and links with the heart. It starts from the outside of the heart, goes upward to arrive at the armpit and then turns around at the shoulder. Traveling downward all the way along the inner arm, it arrives at the center of the palm, and links the tip of the fingers to the palm center. As this meridian travels up and down the arm, its route almost overlaps at the midline of the arm. There is one branch on either side, very easy to find.

While relaxing, you can massage and knead your Pericardium Meridian along its route, up to down, for about 10 minutes. Then change to the other hand. In addition to massaging and kneading it with the hand, we can also tap it with an empty fist all the way along both inner arms. You can tap the meridian before going to bed at night, or when you are relaxing and have free time, with a moderate force.

Please note that if you feel pain or numbness when a spot is pressed, then the meridian at this spot has stagnated and is jammed. Therefore it needs to be massaged and kneaded strongly. Pay more attention to this spot every day by tapping

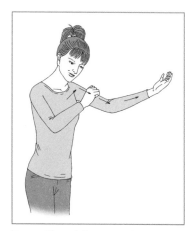

Tap and knead the Pericardium Meridian.

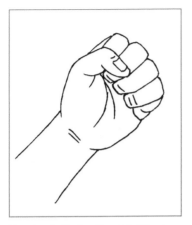

Exercise the Pericardium Meridian by clenching fists.

and kneading it additional times, until the sense of pain or numbness has vanished. Do not treat this lightly, because the heart can be affected and heart diseases occur if the Pericardium Meridian does not run smoothly or is jammed.

While passing the palm, the Pericardium Meridian has two important acupoints, the Zhongchong point and Laogong point. The Zhongchong point is located at the tip of the middle finger. The Laogong point is located between the second and third metacarpal bone of the palm (closer to latter), under the tip of the middle finger when we make a fist and bend our fingers.

Stimulating these two acupoints can strengthen the force of the pericardium. The method is simple, and in fact we often practice this action subconsciously. When feeling nervous, at a loss or angry, we sometimes clench our hand into a fist, which brings on a feeling as if an invisible force has made us quiet down. This is actually an effect of stimulating these two acupoints on the Pericardium Meridian. As a daily practice, we can consciously clench both fists, thus stimulating the Zhongchong and Laogong points, which will exercise our Pericardium Meridian and regulate its function.

Exercising the Pericardium Meridian can effectively protect our heart, and avoid the invasion of diseases of the heart, first among our five important internal organs. A healthy heart can ensure that the other internal organs work systematically, and put us on the road to a healthy, happy and long life.

Chapter Twelve

Hai Time (9 p.m. to 11 p.m.)
Sanjiao Meridian in Its Prime

At Hai Time (9 p.m. to 11 p.m.) all things on the earth are in a quiet state. Yin energy reaches its prime but will begin to wane gradually, and yang energy remains at its weakest but will begin to wax slowly. This is the time leading to the exchange of yin and yang in the heavens and on earth, with a new round of cycle about to begin.

At Hai Time the Shaoyang Sanjiao Meridian of Hand (Sanjiao Meridian) works. The Sanjiao, or "Triple Heater," is an organ specific to TCM, and is comprised of the three parts that span from the thoracic down to the abdominal-pelvic cavities. The Upper Jiao and Middle Jiao are separated by the diaphragm, with the section above (including the heart and lungs) being the Upper Jiao. Below the diaphragm and above the navel (including the spleen and stomach) is the Middle Jiao, and below the navel is the Lower Jiao, including the kidneys, bladder, large intestine, small intestine and uterus.

According to *Yellow Emperor's Inner Canon*, the Sanjiao is in charge of water channels all over our body. As a connector of internal organs, it can help to clear these channels and normally excrete body fluids. In addition to body fluids, the Sanjiao can also operate the vital energy stored in the kidney. The blood and energy needed by the body are transferred and judiciously distributed by the Sanjiao.

When we are dreaming, our body also needs to consume energy. Where does this energy come from? It is transported to our internal organs through the Sanjiao Meridian. The operation of the Sanjiao is regulated through Sanjiao Meridian. Because of this, the Sanjiao Meridian is very important for our health, and we should pay attention to its maintenance and exercise.

Rehabilitate When All Things Are in a Quiet State

At Zi Time (11 p.m. to 1 a.m.) and Wu Time (11 a.m. to 1 p.m.), we can reach the best quality of sleep. Moreover it is prime time for nourishing our yin and yang. We should start our journey toward good sleep at Hai Time.

At noon, a half-hour nap can replenish yang energy, thus making sure that we have enough vital essence to face the afternoon. However we need to sleep for a long time at night, especially at Zi Time. This is the golden time for sleep, a time when we should be in a state of deep sleep.

According to *Yellow Emperor's Inner Canon*, at Zi Time (midnight), yin energy reaches its peak and then begins to wane, while yang energy is at almost zero but beginning to build. The yin and yang in the heavens and on earth are exchanged. As this exchange between yin and yang reaches its maximum, we can nourish yin by sleeping soundly. However it is always difficult to reach a state of sound sleep

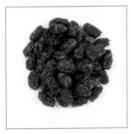

Chinese Dates

all at once. For centuries people have looked at sleep as a step-by-step process, and as tradition holds, "We should put our eyes to sleep before putting our heart to sleep."

At Hai Time we can close our eyes, calm our mind, and naturally bring ourselves into the state of sleep, so that we are able to fall into deep sleep at Zi Time.

If you often suffer from bad sleep or insomnia, it is recommended to take up some gentle activities before sleep, such as listening to some light and soft music, watching relaxing television programs, or even just sitting still on a sofa. You can also eat some special sleep-promoting items, including yin-tonifying and energy-replenishing food such as Chinese-date porridge, lotus root starch, sweet soup of lily bulb and lotus seed, or a glass of warm milk.

In addition, bathing the feet is effective for relieving fatigue and promoting sleep, especially for middle-aged and older people. It can promote coordination between the heart and kidneys. This coordination enables the mutual aid of water and heat, which can promote coordination between yin and yang. This allows our state of sleep to be optimal.

Sleep and food are the most important considerations for health preservation. Proper sleep can replenish energy and restore vigor, with the effect of nourishing yin and cultivating vital essence. Therefore we should always make sleep a priority.

Successfully Fight the Clock after 35

In terms of health, after the age of 35, various functions of the human body begin to decline, with the speed of aging increasing. Immortality is impossible, because it goes against the laws of Mother Nature. However changes in our daily habits can help slow down our aging. These can be simple things such as going to bed before 11 p.m. every night. If we can persist in doing this, then it is not impossible to retain youthful characteristics, even after 35.

However, regrettably, nowadays few people can do this completely. The period around the age of 35 is often when people are at the busiest point in their life, in terms of career and family. At this time most people are on a definite career track, and to advance they often work overtime every day, and return home late, beginning another day's work after sleeping for only a few hours. They also need to support their family, sometimes both children and parents.

Therefore, with this mental stress and long-term high pressure, it is no surprise that for many people the quality of their sleep is poor, and few of them go to sleep before 11 p.m. This has consequences on health, and early-aging becomes an inevitable result. Therefore it is not surprising that their skin worsens, wrinkles appear, and their hair turns grey. This is caused by long-term inattention to proper sleep.

The Sanjiao Meridian is in its prime at Hai Time. As we have seen, it is in charge of transporting and deploying vital energy and body fluids. If we do anything other than sleeping at this time, too much vital essence and blood becomes concentrated at one place in the body, and the Sanjiao Meridian is unable to allocate enough energy to other places.

Without enough "food supply," other tissues in the body will "complain" and "protest," causing problems over the long run. If the Sanjiao Meridian does not work properly, sweat and urine are not excreted normally, thus resulting in endocrine disorders. Therefore we should go to sleep at Hai Time, helping to maintain normal excretion and to promote metabolism.

TCM states that the Sanjiao is interlinked with all channels. When the energy and blood that can be deployed by the Sanjiao are sufficient, the various channels run smoothly. When energy and blood are plentiful, pathological factors will not invade. If we go to sleep at Hai Time every day, our Sanjiao Meridian can function optimally, nourishing all channels in our body and dispensing with waste. Then we will find no disease and pain in any part of the body, and we will naturally feel and look younger.

Keep Hands and Feet Warm

In winter most people, especially women and older people,

often feel ice-cold in their hands and feet. Even if they wear thick thermal clothes or stay in a heated room, their hands and feet still feel very cold, sometimes to the point of pain. Why?

According to traditional Chinese medicine, there is insufficient yang energy in the body in winter. Since little yang energy is delivered to our hands and feet, we will feel a sense of cold there. In addition, when the air temperature is low in winter, the blood vessels shrink and the back-flow ability of the blood also declines. Therefore since the blood circulation in the hands and feet is not regular, the feeling of coldness will persist there. We can solve this problem by regulating our Yangchi point and bathing our feet.

The Yangchi point is easy to find, because it is located at the joint of the bones at the back of the hands. To find it stretch out your hand, slightly raise the back of your hand, and several creases will occur on your wrist. At the center you will discover a fossula, or small pit. This point is the exact location of the Yangchi point.

Near the wrist and ankle, twelve meridians and collaterals each have a respective source acupoint for the passage and concentration of vital essence. The source acupoint of the Sanjiao Meridian is the Yangchi point. Massaging and practicing moxibustion on the Yangchi point can improve the symptom of cold hands and feet.

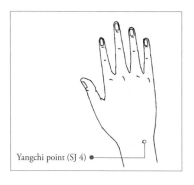

Yangchi point (SJ 4) ●

The Yangchi point is where the vital energy of the Sanjiao Meridian passes through and gathers in the hands.

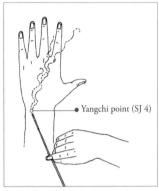

Practicing moxibustion on the Yangchi point regulates energy and blood circulation in the entire Sanjiao Meridian.

Massaging Method

Rubbing the backs of both hands to produce heat, press the Yangchi point of one hand with the middle finger of the other, for 10 to 15 minutes. Then change your hands and repeat the action on the other hand. Apply a moderate force.

Moxibustion

For the hands: Igniting a moxa stick, put it about 2 cm away from the Yangchi point, for about 15 to 20 minutes consistently every day. When a lot of yang energy gathers here, it is naturally conducted to your fingers, and your hands will become hot. After two months the symptom of coldness in the hands should show obvious improvement. In addition, stimulating this source acupoint on the Sanjiao Meridian can promote the energy and blood circulation of the entire meridian.

For the feet: We can improve cold feet by bathing them. First prepare some moxa leaves, and put them in water, heating until boiling. Then bathe your feet in the water. Take care that the water temperature is kept within a range that makes you feel a little hot in your feet. You can add hot water at any time when the water cools. Bathe your feet about 20 minutes at a time. It is best to go directly to bed after bathing. After a month of this practice the symptoms should be improved.

People with cold hands and feet should practice the above methods preferably at Hai Time. Since the Sanjiao Meridian is in its prime, and energy and blood flow past it, regulating the meridian at this time produces a better curative effect. Although the method is important, the key still lies in persistence. Only continual practice can thoroughly eliminate the symptoms of cold hands and feet.

Regulate Sanjiao Meridian to Help with Climacteric Syndromes

In women the transitional period from middle age to old age is called menopause. A relatively outstanding feature of menopausal women can be uncontrollable and changeable moods. They tend to become irritable over small matters, take things unduly seriously, and often feel much regret after losing their temper. Some women are gloomy and indifferent, unwilling to communicate with others, and even depressive. Some are suspicious and apprehensive, always suspecting their husbands of affairs, thus affecting their conjugal relationship.

In TCM all problems related to emotions have something to do with the Sanjiao Meridian. Problems occurring in female climacteric period, the decline in fertility ending in menopause, can be solved by regulating the Sanjiao Meridian.

This meridian is in charge of vital energy, serving as its controller all over the body, and dealing with all problems with vital energy. In the climacteric period, obvious physiological changes happen to women. Ovarian function declines gradually, endocrine disorders occur, and various organs and the nervous system age more and more rapidly.

These physiological changes produce a huge psychological impact upon women, thus leading to obvious changes of mood. These mood changes certainly produce a kind of energy. If this kind of energy is too strong, it accelerates blood flow. When too much energy and blood arrive in the heart, the heart beats faster, and moods become irritable and nervous.

On the contrary, if women forcibly suppress their anger to prevent this kind of energy from being vented, the energy becomes a kind of redundant energy in the body, i.e. the so-called "internal heat." Since there is no normal way for this heat to be vented, it becomes like an uncontrollable wild horse dashing around madly in the body.

When the redundant heat goes into the head, it causes headache; when it goes into the four limbs, it causes rheumatism. This is why climacteric females often suffer from headache and dizziness. The excess energy in the body needs to be controlled and suppressed by a strong force. The Sanjiao Meridian plays this precise role.

All energy and blood in the body are reasonably distributed by the Sanjiao Meridian, so that they do not become overly concentrated at a certain place, such as the liver and heart. If redundant energy is evenly scattered to various corners of the body, no negative effect will occur.

Another function of the Sanjiao is governing the excretion of all body fluids including urine and sweat. In addition to the obvious changes of mood, involuntary hot flashes and perspiration often happen to women in the climacteric period. Excess perspiration is a manifestation of endocrine dyscrasia. Since the Sanjiao Meridian is in charge of endocrine disorders, we can improve this condition by dredging this meridian.

There are many methods for curing climacteric syndromes, and women at this period of their life should take care of their Sanjiao Meridian on a daily basis. In fact it is not a horrible thing for women to enter their climacteric period, which is a natural change in life. They should cherish a positive attitude and should face their life optimistically. It is also beneficial if people around them offer more understanding and support.

How to Exercise the Sanjiao Meridian

The Shaoyang Sanjiao Meridian of Hand, namely the Sanjiao Meridian, starts from the Guanchong point located at ulnar end of the ring finger. It goes upward along the ulnar edge of the ring finger, and passes the Zhongzhu and Yangchi points on the back of the hand. Traveling further upward between the two bones (ulna and radius) on the extensor side of the upper arm, it passes the elbow, reaches the outer side of the upper arm, and moves upward to reach the shoulder. It then crosses behind the Shaoyang Gallbladder Meridian of Foot, enters the supraclavicular fossa, and connects with the pericardium at the Danzhong point of the Conception Vessel. It goes downward, passes the diaphragm, and becomes part of the Sanjiao from the chest to the abdomen.

Its branch goes upward from the chest, traveling out from the supraclavicular fossa, and then upward, passing the neck. It goes upward along the back of the ear, arrives at the frontal angle, and then bends and goes downward along the cheek, arriving at the lower part of the eye socket.

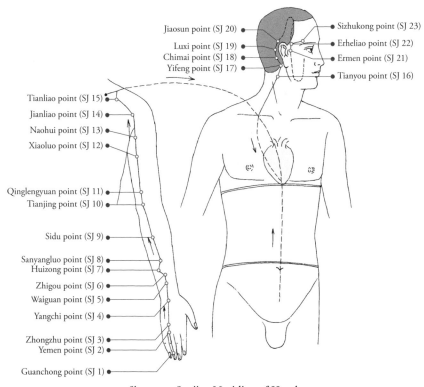

Shaoyang Sanjiao Meridian of Hand

The other branch enters the ear from the back of the ear, goes out and moves in front of the ears. It crosses the first branch at the cheek, arrives at the outer corner of the eye, and links with the Shaoyang Gallbladder Meridian of Foot.

In the outer arm, the Shaoyang Sanjiao Meridian of Hand can be exercised by tapping, preferably between 9 p.m. and 11 p.m. At this time, when the Sanjiao Meridian is in its prime with the most energy and blood, exercising has the best effect.

According to TCM, the Sanjiao is interlinked with all channels. If we regulate and nourish this meridian as part of our daily routine, the blood and energy in all channels of our body will run smoothly, blocking any pathological factors from entering.

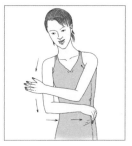

Tap the Sanjiao Meridian.

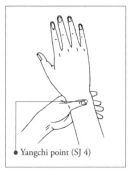

Yangchi point (SJ 4)

Massage the Yangchi point.

Tapping the Sanjiao Meridian

The exercise method is simple. Standing or sitting, tap the outer arm with the other hand all the way down to the wrist, along the route of the Sanjiao Meridian. Use a slightly strong force, for about 10 minutes. Then press and knead the Yangchi point at the back of hand for about three minutes. After that, change to the other hand and use the same method.

Massaging the Yangchi Point

The Yangchi point is like a small barrier. Frequently pressing and kneading this acupoint can guide the energy and blood in the Sanjiao out to the fingers, thus promoting the smooth operation and blood circulation of the entire meridian.

Appendices

Basics of Meridians and Acupuncture Points

According to traditional Chinese medicine, acupuncture points are tiny spots where qi and blood are infused in meridians, collaterals and internal organs. They are not only reaction points of diseases, but also stimulation points for acupuncture, moxibustion and other treatment.

Inside the human body, there are 12 "regular" meridian and collateral channels in total. Adding in the Conception Vessel at the front center of the body and the Governing Vessel at the rear center, there are together fourteen meridian and collateral channels. A total of 365 acupuncture points are arranged along them.

In naming meridians/collaterals and acupuncture points, this books uses codes from the standard of World Federation of Chinese Medicine Societies—Specialty Committee of Publishers and Editors, namely: abbreviations of meridian/collateral names plus serial numbers. For acupuncture point names, Chinese pinyin names (transliterated names) are used.

This book also lists the locations of acupuncture points so that readers can find them conveniently. An important means of location is the "cun" measurements of the body. This system is an ingenious way by which anyone can measure and locate acupoints on his or her own body. Since everyone's body is of a different size and shape, using a measurement system specific to the individual makes finding the points easy.

The process starts with the measurement of one cun. This is done in two ways:

- Using the width of the distal inter-phalangeal joint of the thumb.
- Using the distance between the distal and proximal inter-phalangeal joints of the third (middle) finger.

All other specific measurements are outlined in the diagrams below. When in doubt in measuring, the thumb (1 cun) or the four finger method (3 cun) can always be used.

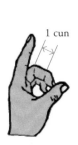

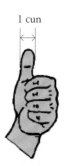

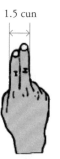

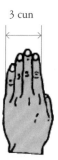

1 cun   1 cun   1.5 cun   3 cun

Standard Meridian Abbreviations

Taiyin Lung Meridian of Hand ···································· LU
Yangming Large Intestine Meridian of Hand ··············· LI
Yangming Stomach Meridian of Foot ························· ST
Taiyin Spleen Meridian of Foot ······························ SP
Shaoyin Heart Meridian of Hand ···························· HT
Taiyang Small Intestine Meridian of Hand ················· SI
Taiyang Bladder Meridian of Foot ·························· BL
Shaoyin Kidney Meridian of Foot ·························· KI
Jueyin Pericardium Meridian of Hand ····················· PC
Shaoyang Sanjiao Meridian of Hand ······················· SJ
Shaoyang Gallbladder Meridian of Foot ···················· GB
Jueyin Liver Meridian of Foot ······························ LV
Conception Vessel ·· RN
Governing Vessel ··· DU
Extra Points of the Head and Neck ······················ EX-HN

Index